Assitan Kolé COULIBALY
Fatogoma Issa KONE
Mohamed Amadou KEITA

Management of Post-Thyroidectomy Recurrent Paralysis

Assitan Kolé COULIBALY
Fatogoma Issa KONE
Mohamed Amadou KEITA

Management of Post-Thyroidectomy Recurrent Paralysis

Post-thyroidectomy recurrent paralysis

ScienciaScripts

Imprint

Cover image: www.ingimage.com

This book is a translation from the original published under ISBN 978-620-6-70593-2.

Publisher:
Sciencia Scripts
is a trademark of
Dodo Books Indian Ocean Ltd. and OmniScriptum S.R.L publishing group

120 High Road, East Finchley, London, N2 9ED, United Kingdom
Str. Armeneasca 28/1, office 1, Chisinau MD-2012, Republic of Moldova, Europe
Printed at: see last page
ISBN: 978-620-8-07047-2

Contents

Working together:

Dr Naouma Cissé

Dr Ibrahim Dicko

Acknowledgements :

- Professor kadidiatou Sangaré
- Professor Soumaoro Siaka
- Professor Boubacary Guindo
- Dr Kassim Diarra
- Dr N'Faly Konaté
- Dr Kalifa Coulibaly
- To all the DES in the ENT department

INTRODUCTION

Recurrent paralysis is dysfunction of one or both of the lower laryngeal nerves, most often resulting in paralysis of the intrinsic muscles of the larynx which are innervated by the lower laryngeal nerves(1).

Post-thyroidectomy recurrent paralysis (RP) is the most frequent and most feared complication. It occurs following injury to the recurrent nerve in 26 to 59% of cases(2). The anatomical proximity of the recurrent nerve to the thyroid gland increases the risk of recurrent paralysis.

This complication was described with high rates from the early days of thyroid surgery and was responsible for many deaths. The high rate of this complication at the outset quickly led to a change in surgical technique, with the nerves being located intraoperatively or an intra capsular dissection being performed, with some success. Since then, the risk has diminished, but it persists and must always be reported (3).

It may be unilateral, causing dysphonia, or bilateral, resulting in laryngeal dyspnoea on extubation(3) , which may be life-threatening.

The incidence of recurrent complications of the laryngeal nerve in African and international literature is currently between 2 and 6%(5). The incidence of post-thyroidectomy recurrent paralysis was 1.5 to 5.3% according to the study by Hung-Chun Chen et al, of which 15% to 17% were cases of permanent vocal cord paralysis(6).

Over a ten-year period, Lamia Dbab found 1,000 patients with thyroid pathology operated on, representing an average of 100 thyroidectomies per year. Of these patients, 750 underwent total thyroidectomy and 250 hemi thyroidectomy, representing 1,750 recurrent nerves located and dissected. 12 cases (1.2%) of postoperative unilateral RA were recorded during this period; no case of bilateral RA was observed (4).

A review of the literature highlights the rarity of cases of bilateral paralysis, with 0.4% according to Rosato (7).

Various devices have been described to reduce the frequency of this complication, but it seems that the essential rule is to follow a careful, rigorous and standardised surgical technique, including locating the recurrent nerve (4) .

They pose a serious problem for ear, nose and throat specialists. In the past, the treatment of this condition was based on transcervical surgery of the arytenoid since 1922, but today there have been many advances with the advent of endoscopic laser treatment since Ossof's arytenoidectomy (8).

In Mali, recurrent lesions accounted for 2.8% of complications in 158 thyroidectomies performed over a period of 5 years and were transient (9). The management of recurrent lesions is a problem in our context because of the investigations required to initiate appropriate management. The impact on socio-professional and educational quality of life in the case of bilateral paralysis must be emphasised, and its management requires a compromise between phonation and respiration. Based on previous studies on the management of recurrent paralysis, our aim in this study was to evaluate our experience and compare the results with those in the literature.

OBJECTIVES

> GENERAL OBJECTIVE

- To describe the epidemiological, diagnostic and therapeutic aspects of post-thyroidectomy recurrent paralysis.

> SPECIFIC OBJECTIVES

- To determine the frequency of post-thyroidectomy recurrent paralysis according to socio-demographic characteristics.
- Analyse the various diagnostic aspects.
- List the risk factors for post-thyroidectomy recurrent paralysis.
- Evaluate our experience in managing this complication.

CHAPTER I

GENERAL

II.REMINDERS

1. ANATOMICAL REMINDERS

1.1.ANATOMICAL OVERVIEW OF THE THYROID GLAND(10)

In physiological terms, the thyroid is roughly butterfly-shaped. Its two lateral lobes are joined at the front by the thyroid isthmus, with a median pyramidal lobe - or pyramid of La Louette - which is superior and inconstant. It is situated in the mid-cervical position, in front of the larynx and trachea, with the isthmus opposite the second and third tracheal rings and the upper poles flush with the thyroid cartilage.

Below, the lower pole responds - head hyperextended - to the fifth or sixth tracheal ring.

The thyroid cavity is defined anteriorly by the subhyoid muscles, laterally by the sternocleidomastoid muscles and deep down by the aerodigestive axes, with the thyroid moulding itself to the larynx and trachea anteriorly and to the oesophagus posteriorly, and by the cervical vascular and neural axes posterolaterally: common carotid artery medially, internal jugular vein laterally, vagus nerve in the posterior dihedron.

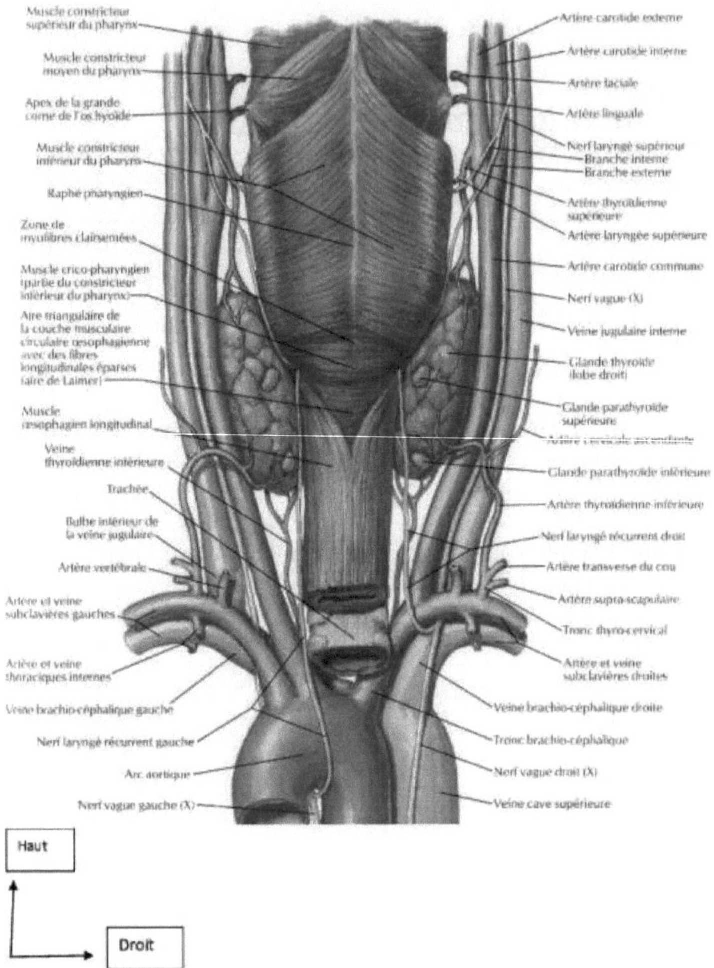

Figure 1: Posterior view of the neck showing important relationships (11)

1.2. ANATOMY OF THE LARYNX :

1.2.1. EXTERNAL CONFIGURATION OF THE LARYNX: (11-14)

The larynx is a musculo-cartilaginous airway located in the middle and anterior part of the neck, in front of the hypopharynx below the hyoid bone and above the trachea (vertebral body from C4 to the lower edge of C6). Its structure is mainly cartilaginous, made up of five (05) main cartilages:

- Thyroid cartilage ;
- The cricoid cartilage ;
- The arytenoid cartilages (two in number) ;
- Epiglottic cartilage.

> **Thyroid cartilage** :
The most voluminous, it is the protective part of the larynx. The cartilage is made up of two quadrangular blades, forming a dihedral angle open at the back and responsible, at the front, for the relief of the laryngeal prominence or ADAM's apple.

> **The cricoid cartilage :**
It is the essential element of the framework: It is the base. It is located in the lower part of the larynx and is shaped like a signet ring with a posterior bezel measuring 2 cm high on a ring or anterior arch measuring approximately 5 mm high.

> **The arytenoid cartilages :**
The arytenoid cartilage is shaped like a pyramid, the base of which articulates with the cricoid. There are two of them, located above the cricoid chaton and behind the thyroid cartilage. They are described as having three faces:

> An internal submucosal surface ;

> A posterior face, and
- One anterolateral side.
The arytenoid cartilages play a fundamental role in laryngeal physiology thanks to two types of movement: a sliding or translational movement: by sliding forwards, the two arytenoids move away from each other and the glottis opens; by sliding backwards they move towards each other, causing the glottis to close; movements of anterior rotation around a vertical axis passing through the centre of the articular surfaces.

> **The epiglottic cartilage :**
It is shaped like a snowshoe or flower petal, with a posterior-inferior laryngeal surface facing downwards and backwards and a concave anterosuperior lingual surface facing upwards and forwards. Between the base of the tongue and the anterior (lingual or pharyngeal) surface of the epiglottis is the vallecula. These different elements of the laryngeal cartilage are joined by membranes and ligaments, the most important of which is the thyroartenoid ligament or vocal cord ligament. The muscles allow the larynx to be mobile, particularly during swallowing and breathing.
From a morphological point of view, the larynx should be considered as an elastic tube reinforced by the cricoid and arytenoids, attached to the median part of the thyroid-hyoid apparatus. It is angled, narrowed in the middle and protrudes into the pharynx in the form of a cylinder which is swollen in the lower part and bevelled in the upper part in a plane which slopes downwards and backwards. It is lined by a mucosa continuous with the pharyngeal and tracheal mucosa, and lined by a fibroelastic membrane stretched from the epiglottic ligament Ary at the top to the cricoid arch at the bottom.

1.2.2. THE INTERNAL CONFIGURATION OF THE LARYNX (14-16)

The larynx is a 5 cm high tube, 3.5 cm wider at the top. The laryngeal mucosa is of the respiratory type and continues above, beyond the glosso-epiglottic groove with the basi-lingual mucosa: it is cleavable on the anterior surface of the epiglottis. It is lined by a mucosa continuous with the pharyngeal and tracheal mucosa. This mucosa is lined by a fibroelastic membrane stretched from the epiglottic ligament Ary at the top to the cricoid arch at the bottom.

- **The fibroelastic membrane has two thickenings:**
- The vestibular or superior thyroartenoid ligament, stretched between the re-entrant angle of the thyroid and the arytenoid cartilage;
- The vocal ligament or inferior thyroartenoid ligament, stretched between the re-entrant angle of the thyroid and the vocal process of the arytenoid cartilage.
- **The fibroelastic membrane is divided into three segments by these ligaments:**
- Upper segment, forming the quadrangular membrane above the vestibular ligament;
- Middle segment: the elastic cone or membrane invaginates to form the ventricle of Morgagni's larynx, which has an anterior diverticulum, the laryngeal saccule;
- Lower segment, below the vocal ligament.
- **The laryngeal cavity is divided into three levels by two folds:**

The upper vocal cords or vestibular folds, subtended by the lateral thyroarytenoid muscle and the superior thyroarytenoid ligament;

The lower vocal cords, underpinned by the ligament and vocal muscle, bound the glottis cleft between them.

The three stages of the larynx are :

- **The upper stage or laryngeal vestibule**, bounded at the top by the laryngeal aditus and at the bottom by the vestibular cleft between the vestibular folds;
- **The middle stage**, glottic stage, vocal cords and arytenoids;
- **The lower or infraglottic stage**, which is continuous with the trachea at the bottom.

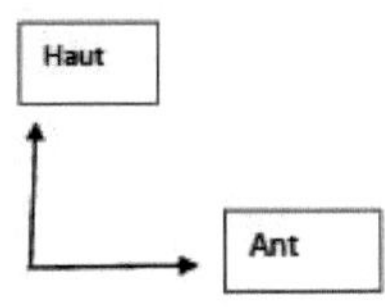

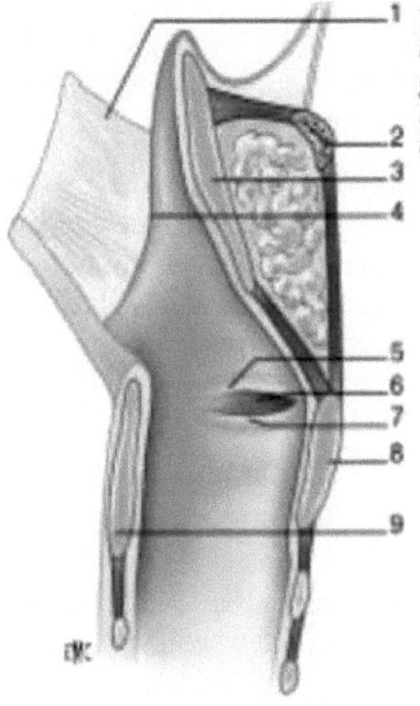

1. Membrane thyrohyoïdienne ; 2. os hyoïde ; 3. épiglotte ; 4. repli aryténoépiglottique ; 5. bande ventriculaire ; 6. ventricule de Morgagni ; 7. corde vocale ; 8. cartilage thyroïde ; 9. cartilage cricoïde.

1. Ihyrohyoid Membnine; 2. hyoid bone; **3.** *epiglottis; 4. arytenoepi-glottic fold;* **5.** *ventricular band; 6. Morgagni's ventricle;* **7.** *vocal cord; 8. thyroid cartilage; 9. elicoid cartilage.*

Figure 2: Sagittal section of the larynx((14)

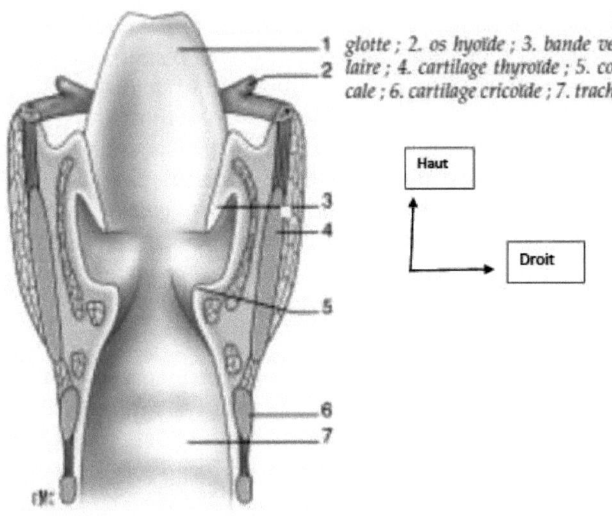

1. *Epi-*

1 *glottis; 2 hyoid bone;* **3** *ventricular band; 2* **4** *thyroid cartilage;* **5** *vocal cord; 6 cricoid cartilage; 7 trachea.*

Figure 3: Frontal section of the larynx (14)

1.2.2.1. The vocal cord :

The vocal cord or vocal fold is made up of several histological layers. The structure of the vocal cords should be considered as a superposition of several layers of different viscosity and elasticity (from surface to depth: the epithelium, the lamina propria itself separated into three layers, and the vocal muscle) (17).

> **Epithelium**

The vocal cords are covered by non-keratinised stratified squamous epithelium. Its distinctive feature is the absence of mucous glands at the free edge. Moisture is provided by mucus secreted by adjacent areas. The basal epithelial layer is firmly anchored to the submucosal layer by anchoring proteins in the basement membrane. The epithelium, 0.05-0.1mm thick, encapsulates the more fluid tissue of the submucosa like a "balloon full of water" (18).

> **Lamina propria (submucosa)**

This is the structure mainly responsible for cord vibration. It is made up of three layers: superficial, intermediate and deep. The superficial lamina propria is immediately submucosal. It corresponds to Reinke's space (15).

Its properties of suppleness and extensibility are essential to ensure harmonious propagation of the vibratory wave. It is made up of few collagen fibres, which are short and not very dense, and a few fine, longitudinal elastic fibres, which are adapted to longitudinal stretching stresses (17). It contains numerous proteoglycans which give it its viscous properties (17). The intermediate and deep layers make up the vocal ligament, which supports the vibration. The intermediate layer is made up of thicker, anteroposteriorly oriented elastic fibres; the deep layer is essentially made up of dense collagen fibres (14). Tissue repair in this layer is more uncertain than in the superficial layer, as the architecture and orientation of the collagen fibres are often disrupted. Damage to these layers by pathology or extensive surgery therefore leads to significant disruption of vibration (14). To avoid confusing them with cystic formations, surgeons should also be aware of the existence of macula flavae (18). These are reinforcements of the vocal ligament responsible for localised thickening at the anterior and posterior levels of the vocal cords, where the mechanical stresses are greatest. Most of the protein and cell synthesis and renewal of the vocal ligament takes place within these macula flavae(18).

> **Vocal muscle**

This is the thyroarytenoid muscle, a striated muscle innervated by the inferior laryngeal nerve. Its boundary with the vocal ligament is barely visible due to the numerous exchanges of fibres between the two structures. The biomechanical properties of the vocal cord vary according to the degree of contraction of the thyroarytenoid muscle(19).

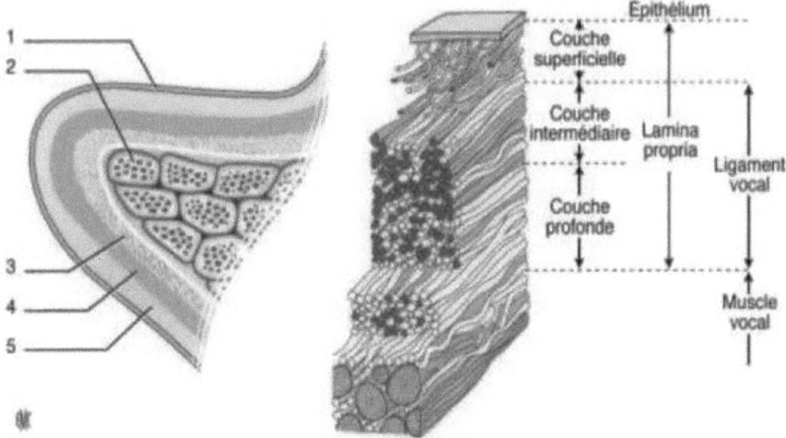

Figure 4: Stratified anatomy of the vocal cord(19)

It is traditional to describe from surface to depth: the epithelium "1", Reinke's space (superficial layer of the lamina propria) "2", the vocal ligament (middle and deep layers of the lamina propria) "3 and 4", the vocal muscle (inferior thyroarytenoid muscle) "5", according to Hirano (19).

1.2.2.2. Innervation

The cord innervation is mixed: sensitive with the superior laryngeal nerve, and motor with the recurrent nerves(11).

1.3. ANATOMY OF THE RECURRENT NERVES

The recurrent or inferior laryngeal nerve is the motor nerve of the larynx. It is a collateral branch of the vagus or vagus nerve, the tenth cranial pair (X). The right and left recurrent nerves have different anatomy (4).

1.3.1. Right recurrent nerve: (4)

> **Origin:** Detaches from the X at the superior border of the right subclavian artery and describes a pre-, sub- and retroarterial arch above the pleural dome.

> **Journey and reports :**

Unlike the left recurrent nerve, the right recurrent nerve has a purely cervical course. It ascends in the cellular tissue of the visceral lodge of the neck, obliquely anteriorly and medially, towards the crico-thyroid gutter. It crosses the posterior surface of the primitive carotid artery, then lies medial to it (sub-thyroid segment). It crosses the right edge of the oesophagus to reach the posterior edge of the trachea. Outside the subthyroid artery, the inferior thyroid artery rises parallel to the subthyroid artery in the lymph node tissue (Gougenheim's recurrent chain). The retrothyroidal portion is in close contact with the posteromedial surface of the thyroid lobe, which is attached to the first 2-3 tracheal rings by Grüber's ligament, in which it is embedded. It then passes in front of the horizontal segment or between the branches of the inferior thyroid artery. The inferior parathyroid is 1-2cm outside the artery-nerve crossing. The right recurrent nerve forms a crossover with an internal concavity and engages under the inferior bundle of the inferior constrictor, in the crico-thyroid gutter. This intra-laryngeal penetration point is located at the level of the small horn of the thyroid cartilage.

> **Termination:** The left recurrent nerve terminates intra-laryngeally in two posterior and anterior branches. The posterior branch, on the external surface of the crico-arytenoid muscles, forms Gallien's loop, anastomosing with the superior laryngeal muscle and giving branches to the posterior crico-arytenoid muscle, which is the only dilator of the vocal cords, and to the intrearytenoid muscle. The anterior branch with branches to the lateral crico-arytenoid and thyro-arytenoid muscles.

1.3.2. Left recurrent nerve: (4)

> **Origin:** Thoracic branch of the left vagus nerve, from which it detaches at the anterolateral aspect of the aortic arch.

> **Journey and reports :**

- **At its origin:** it lies between the inferior surface of the aorta and the anterosuperior surface of the left main branch, outside the arterial ligament.
- **In the thoracic portion,** the nerve travels upwards along the anterior wall of the oesophagus, which extends posteriorly beyond the posterior edge of the trachea, which is laterally deviated to the right. The left primitive carotid artery lies in an anterior plane.
- **In its cervical portion:** the nerve remains pre-oesophageal and laterotracheal at the base of the neck, surrounded by cellulo-ganglionic tissue. It is crossed laterally by the arch of the thoracic duct. The recurrent remains posterior to the vascular bundle of the neck formed by the primitive carotid artery covered by the brachiocephalic venous trunk.
- **In its sub-thyroid segment:** the nerve remains behind and medial to the inferior thyroid artery within a cellular tissue containing Gougenheim's recurrent ganglion chain.
- **The nerve is then retrothyroid:** remaining behind the inferior thyroid artery, it is posterior to Grüber's ligament which attaches the thyroid lobe to the 2nd and 3rd tracheal rings. The inferior parathyroid lies behind the recurrent.
- **Above Grüber's ligament:** the recurrent forms a crossover at the base.

It enters under the inferior constrictor of the pharynx to reach the crico-thyroid gutter. This point of penetration is marked by the small horn of the thyroid cartilage. This is the most difficult area to dissect.

> **Termination:** The left recurrent nerve terminates intra-laryngeally in two posterior and anterior branches. The posterior branch, on the external surface of the cricoarytenoid muscles, forms Gallien's loop, anastomosing with the superior laryngeal muscle and giving branches to the posterior cricoarytenoid muscle, which is the only dilator of the vocal cords, and to the inter-arytenoid muscle. The anterior branch with branches to the lateral cricoarytenoid and thyroarytenoid muscles.

1.3.3. COLLATERAL BRANCHES :

Each laryngeal nerve gives :

- Tracheal frames ,
- Heart attacks
- Pharyngeal frames
- And oesophageal branches

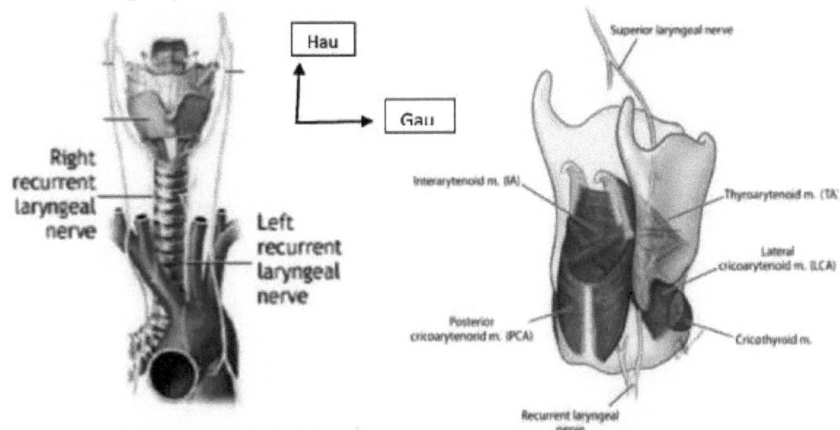

Figure 5: Origin and termination of the recurrent nerve(17)

1.3.4. ANATOMICAL VARIATIONS :

1.3.4.1. EXTERNAL LARYNGEAL NERVE :

The course of the external laryngeal nerve varies widely. Cernea and Friedman have drawn up classifications of the risk of injury depending on the course of the nerve, making it possible to distinguish between high-risk situations (10).

The Cernea classification (a-c on the diagram) classifies the course of the nerve according to its relationship to the superior thyroid artery and the superior pole of the thyroid body. It was published specifically to classify the risk of injury to the external laryngeal nerve during thyroid surgery. Types IIA (crossing of the artery less than 1 cm above the upper pole) and IIB (crossing of the artery below the level of the upper pole) are considered to be the most at risk of injury to the external laryngeal nerve, even though they account for more than 3 quarters of intra-operative anatomical findings (10).

Friedman's classification (d-f) is based on the relationship between the external laryngeal nerve and the inferior pharyngeal constrictor muscle. In type 1, the nerve is superficial all the way to laryngeal penetration, in type 2 it penetrates the muscle at its lower end, and at its upper end in type 3. Type 1s are obviously the most at risk during thyroid surgery (10).

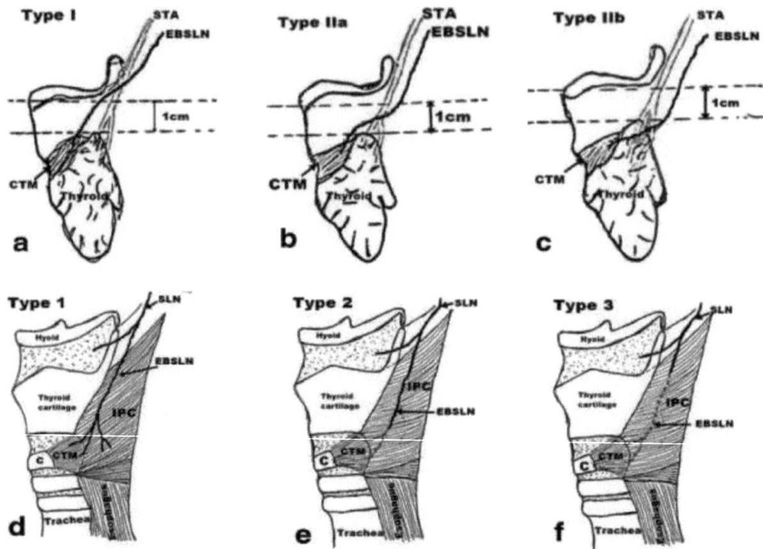

Figure 6: Types of anatomical variants of the external laryngeal nerve (10)

1.3.4.2. RECURRENT NERVE :

The recurrent nerve is characterised by major anatomical variations, particularly on the right side, and there is a risk of injury in 20% of cases (20).

> RELATIONSHIP BETWEEN THE NERVE AND THE ATI :

As for the recurrent nerves, they also vary greatly in their course, with only their origin and termination being fixed (10).

The course of the recurrent nerve is often described in terms of its relationship to the inferior thyroid artery and its branches. All modes of crossing are possible, as shown in the diagram below based on Echeverria Monares "f" (10).

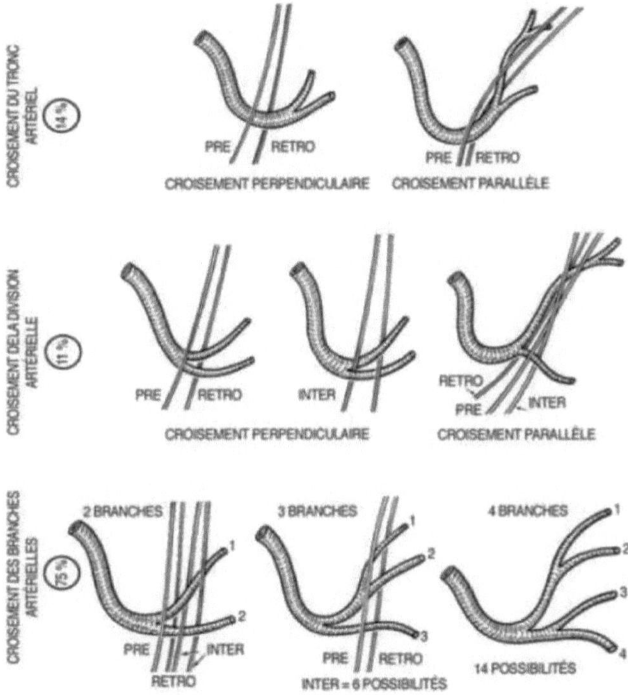

Figure 7: Relationship of the recurrent nerve to the inferior thyroid artery (10)

> **NON-RECURRENT RECURRENT NERVE:** (20)

It should be noted that a non-recurrent recurrent nerve may be abnormal, but without any functional repercussions, with a nerve which arises in a superior position, does not form a subclavian loop and has a vertical downward course to join the larynx. As this anomaly is often associated with abnormalities in the development of the branchial arches, failure to find the recurrent nerve in its usual position means that a search must be made for associated vascular defects (17).

It is easy to see that this enormous variability means that the nerve has to be identified and then strictly monitored.

It should be noted that the discovery of the nerve pathway is always intraoperative and not preoperative, and therefore any dissection must be cautious until the nerves have been identified and protected under visual control (17).

> **BIFURCATION OF THE RECURRENT NERVE :**

Most treatises describe the inferior laryngeal nerve as an isolated nerve passing through the tracheo-oesophageal gutter and entering the larynx at the level of the crico-thyroid membrane. However, studies have shown that the recurrent nerve is often divided at its crossing point, giving rise to branches with different destinations: oesophageal, pharyngeal or tracheal-laryngeal (21).

2. PHYSIOLOGICAL BACKGROUND

2.1.PHYSIOLOGY OF THE RECURRENT NERVES

The recurrent nerve innervates all the muscles of the larynx, with the exception of the cricothyroid muscle: the glottic constrictors (thyroarytenoid, lateral cricoarytenoid, inter-arytenoid) and the posterior cricoarytenoid (glottic dilator). It is therefore the motor nerve of the vocal cord. It therefore plays a role in breathing, phonation and swallowing (4) .

2.1.1. ROLE OF THE RECURRENT NREF IN BREATHING

-inspiration: the larynx and trachea are lowered and the vocal cords are spread by contraction of the posterior cricoarytenoids (4).

-**On** exhalation, the opposite occurs: the larynx rises and the vocal cords come together (4).

2.1.2. ROLE OF THE RECURRENT NERVE IN PHONATION

The recurrent nerve is the motor nerve of the vocal cord. It innervates the constrictor muscles of the glottis and the only dilator muscle of the glottis: the posterior cricoarytenoid. During vocal emission, which occurs during the exhalation phase, the vocal cords first come together in a closed position, thanks to the arytenoid cartilages. The pressure of the expiratory air column (subglottic pressure) comes up against an obstacle (closure of the cords). It increases and forces the free edges of the cords to spread slightly, allowing a small amount of air, or puff, to pass through. As soon as this puff of air is released, the free edges will move closer together again. The phenomenon is repeated periodically as the subglottic pressure increases again, the cords being closed, creating a new vibration. This is how unilateral RA leads to dysphonia due to the absence of confrontation between the two vocal cords, whereas bilateral RA leads to either adducted RA, which includes Gerhardt's syndrome or Riegel's syndrome, or adducted RA or Ziemsen's syndrome, which can be fatal if not treated urgently (4).

2.1.3. ROLE OF THE RECURRENT NERVE IN SWALLOWING

The epiglottis closes the upper orifice as the larynx rises and presses against the base of the tongue, pushing the epiglottis backwards. The vocal cords come together to close the glottis, preventing food from entering the trachea, while liquids descend into the pharyngolaryngeal gutters (4).

3.REMINDER OF THE THYROIDECTOMY TECHNIQUE :

Thyroid surgery is now fairly standardised, with different stages well described (10).

- Surgery performed under general anaesthetic with orotracheal intubation (10,22).
- Supine position, neck hyperextended (10,22).

3.1.Incision and skin detachment: (22)

The incision must be in a symmetrical Kocher shape, as nothing is more unsightly than an oblique or staggered scar.

The incision must be adapted to each individual case The small approach in principle is not the mark of a great surgeon. The length and position of the

incision depend on the morphology of the neck, the height of the upper poles and the existence of a plunging goitre.
The line of the arched incision, with an upper concavity, is drawn with a dermographic pencil or with the help of a silk thread pressed forcefully into a natural flexion crease of the neck, one or two fingerbreadths above the sternal fork. Generally, the lower the incision, the better the aesthetic result. Two or three scarifications perpendicular to the incision will allow the edges to be accurately coapted during closure.
Access to the cervical lymph nodes must be provided by extending the incision laterally if necessary.
The skin, subcutaneous cellular tissue and skin layer are incised over a length of between 5 and 10 cm.
The upper flap is freed at the surface of the anterior jugular veins and raised beyond the upper edge of the thyroid cartilage. Dissection of certain squint pyramids requires access to the thyroid-hyoid membrane.
The superficial cervical aponeurosis must be respected If the subhyoid muscles are exposed during the elevation of the flap, postoperative adhesions may cause skin fissures during swallowing.If the cervical incision is low, detachment of the Inferior flap up to the upper edge of the sternum is rarely necessary. Laterally, the anterior edge of the sternocleidomastoid is freed by incising the superficial cervical aponeurosis with the hand scalpel or the half-open tip of the scissors, as far as the upper pole of the thyroid body. It is good surgical practice to line the operating field with two small drapes secured with staples.
This minimises the risk of contamination and completes the haemostasis of the section slices.
Exposure can be maintained either by an automatic retractor placed at the upper and lower poles, or by fixing the upper flap to the upper operating field, taking care not to mark the skin of the chin. This can be protected with a compress.

3.2.Exposure of the thyroid cavity:(22)

Good exposure of the thyroid cavity is the best guarantee of quality thyroid surgery. It does not require systematic sectioning of the subhyoid muscles. Lateral reclination of these muscles using Farabeuf retractors allows most goitres to be exposed and freed.
Section of the subhyoid muscles is only necessary in a few special cases:

- Upper pole or nodule very high up and wedged under the insertion of the sternothyroid ;
- Large hypersecretory goitre requiring minimal manipulation of thyroid tissue;
- Thyroid cancer invading the overlying muscle ;
- Incident or operating difficulty requiring rapid action;
- Old goitre with numerous inflammatory flare-ups causing adhesions between the gland and the covering muscles.

The line where the superficial and middle cervical fascia meet is incised with a scalpel from the upper angle of the thyroid cartilage to the sternal fork.
The surgeon and the assistant lift the abutment line on either side using

dissecting forceps, so as to control the opening without any risk of damaging the underlying tissues.
This line, which is said to be white because it is avascular, is in fact crossed by the anastomotic veins of the two anterior jugular veins, which must first be connected. The lateral reclination of the sternocleidohyoid muscles reveals the muscle fibres of the sternothyroid muscles, spread over the superficial surface of the thyroid body. The deep surface of these muscles is detached from the underlying gland using a finger or scissors, then loaded with the long side of the Farabeuf retractor. Traditionally, the space between the sternothyroid and thyroid body that can be detached is avascular, occupied by fine fibrous tracts arranged like a spider's web, which become taut as the detachment progresses and are easily torn. However, it is not uncommon to see fine vessels stretching between the thyroid gland and the deep surface of the sternothyroid muscles. It is vital to identify and coagulate these vessels to avoid unexpected postoperative haematoma. This detachment must be carried through to the outer edge of the gland. In cases of invasive thyroid pathology, the deep surface of the subhyoid muscles may adhere to the thyroid lobes. In these cases, the subhyoid muscles of the thyroid gland are not dissected. They are sectioned above and below the areas of adhesion and are resected in one piece with the thyroid gland. This procedure may encounter an important, albeit inconstant, obstacle: the middle thyroid vein, which drains directly into the internal jugular vein.
Careful ligation frees up the outer edge of the gland as far as the tracheo-oesophageal axis. In the cases mentioned above where the subhyoid muscles must be sectioned, the following technical points must be observed:

- Muscle section must be staggered in relation to the skin incision, and is only performed after the deep surface of the muscles has been cleared, in order to avoid injury to the often dilated subcapsular thyroid vessels, or even a nearby internal jugular vein.
- This section involves the superficial cervical aponeurosis, the anterior jugular vein, the sternocleidohyoid, omohyoid and sternothyroid (whose fibres are often dilated by the expansion of the goitre); the anterior jugular veins will first be bound by transfixing stitches;
- This incision must be made high up, opposite the cricoid, so as to avoid the descending branch of the XII, which approaches these muscles in their lower half;
- After haemostasis, the section slices are marked with forceps as they tend to shrink.

3.3.Next time:(22)
They depend on the type of thyroidectomy performed. In all cases, it is preferable to perfectly locate the midline above and below the thyroid isthmus. This is particularly important when a large goitre distorts and displaces the laryngotracheal axis. It is also an opportunity to dissect and examine the pre-laryngeal and pre-tracheal spaces and to send any suspicious adenopathy for extemporaneous anatomopathological examination.

3.4.Closing:(22)

Irrigating the operating bed with lukewarm saline visualises any haemorrhagic sites and facilitates elective haemostasis. The anaesthetist may be asked to perform a few positive pressure ventilations in order to detect occult venous bleeding. Final washing of the thyroidectomy site is carried out using a non-iodised antiseptic. Drainage is not specifically required during thyroid surgery except in cases where the subhyoid muscles have been sectioned and where a large goitre has been resected. One or two suction drains of the Jost-Redon type are then inserted, exiting in the median pre-sternal region or in line with the scar, taking care not to transfix the external jugular vein. These drains are left in place for 2 to 3 days to help evacuate haematomas and allow the various plans to be applied.

Care must be taken when repairing the muscular and fascial areas.

Once cervical hyperextension has been eliminated, the scar is closed with sutures:

- Either from the skin in one or two planes, with separate stitches, to the staples;
- Or intradermal overlock;
- Or by separate subcutaneous absorbable stitches followed by Steri-Strips on the skin placed perpendicular to the scar.

3.5.Different types of thyroidectomy: (22)

The operative steps described above are common to all types of thyroid surgery and, once the anterior surface of the isthmus and lobes have been exposed, all varieties of thyroidectomy are available to the surgeon.

- Lobo-isthmectomies and total thyroidectomies, because they include the essential procedures for any thyroidectomy.
- Thyroidectomy for plunging goitre.
- Lobo-isthmectomies and total thyroidectomies

These two procedures are performed simultaneously, with total thyroidectomy differing from lobo-isthmectomy only in that it is performed bilaterally. The principle is to remove the whole of one or both thyroid lobes with extra capsular ligation.

3.6.Thyroidectomy for plunging goitres: (3)

The recurrent nerve can be difficult to locate in the case of a large goitre with endothoracic extension. Blind finger dissection of the goitre without locating the recurrent nerve significantly increases the risk of trauma to the nerve. In this case, the authors recommend locating the last extra-laryngeal centimetres of the recurrent nerve and performing retrograde dissection to remove the goitre. If the recurrent nerve is transected, a nerve suture should be performed. It is likely that syncinesia will occur without tonotopy being respected. However, persistent motor tone may help to maintain vocal cord tone, thereby preventing atrophy and positioning of the arytenoid. These elements can help to maintain better glottic function. If the recurrent nerve is clamped or ligated, it is essential to free the nerve from these traumas. Nerve suturing is not indicated in this case. Dissection should begin at the superior pole of the gland on the dipping side.

After ligation of the superior pedicle and identification of the external laryngeal nerve, the lobe is mobilised forwards and downwards.

3.7.Locating and dissecting the recurrent nerve:

During surgery, direct visualisation of the inferior laryngeal nerve is considered the gold standard by the majority of surgeons (23). In the American guidelines, three methods of visualisation of the inferior laryngeal nerve are recommended: the lateral, inferior or superior approach(9,24). The lateral approach is the most commonly used for simple thyroidectomies; the thyroid lobe is retracted medially, the middle thyroid vein is individualised and the recurrent nerve is identified at the middle pole. The inferior approach is recommended for revision or goitre surgery. The nerve is located in the tracheo-oesophageal sulcus, where it crosses the ATI. With the superior approach, the recurrent nerve is identified at the point where it passes beneath the inferior pharyngeal constrictor muscle, close to the cricothyroid junction(24). To help the surgeon identify the nerve, intra-operative neuro-stimulation of the inferior laryngeal nerve has been proposed as likely to reduce the risk of recurrent paralysis.

(25) . Using the stimulator retrograde to the area of signal loss enables the location of the lesion to be identified and its mechanism assessed (crushing, coagulation, nerve section). This makes it possible to assess the prognosis for recovery (26). The neurostimulator is particularly useful in difficult or repeat surgery (27). When bilateral dissection of the recurrent nerves is envisaged, it helps to limit the risk of bilateral paralysis and laryngeal diplegia. If paralysis is suspected, it is recommended that surgery should not be continued on the contralateral side (28).

Involvement of the inferior laryngeal nerve increases the risk of contralateral injury from 9 to 17% (29).

However, this technique does not allow the surgeon to be warned in the event of accidental sectioning of the inferior laryngeal nerve (23).

4.DIAGNOSIS AND TREATMENT

4 .1 POSITIVE DIAGNOSIS :

The diagnosis of paresis, paralysis and/or uni- or bilateral sensitivity disorder is simply that of the manifestation of a condition that must be recognised.

In the case of sudden onset, a history of surgery (thoracic, thyroid, cervical) or influenza may be found in the days or weeks before the onset of dysphonia (30).

RA is the most feared complication of thyroid surgery. Bilateral, it can be life-threatening if not treated urgently. Unilateral, it can lead to dysphonia with a risk of socio-professional handicap (3).

4.1.1 CLINICAL

- **QUESTIONING**

The patient's identity: age; sex; profession; place of residence;

- The mode of onset of the first symptom (dysphonia): sudden or progressive
- Evolution mode (intermittent or permanent)
- Duration: acute (<15 days), sub-acute (between 15 days and 03 months),

chronic (>03 months)

- The patient's medical, surgical and family history (look for any history of thyroidectomy).

The main functional signs are :

- Dysphonia: the voice is fatigable, bitonal and hoarse. Sometimes the patient is only seen at the stage of laryngeal dyspnoea.

-Dyspnoea: this is inspiratory and is codified according to the Chevalier Jackson and Pineau classification into four stages of increasing severity, and is made up of 05 parameters: draught, colouration, state of consciousness, pulse and blood pressure.

- Dry cough
- Swallowing disorders
- Hypersialorrhea
- Odynophagia
- Fever

- **Physical examination**

Clinical examination of the neck is systematic. Look for an old thyroidectomy, tracheotomy or lateral cervicotomy scar. Palpation is used to detect a compressive mass, thyroid tumour or cervical adenopathy (30).

Examination of the larynx is essential in the diagnosis of RA, and either LI or nasofibroscopy is performed.

- **Indirect laryngoscopy (IL):**(31) which most of the time allows a diagnostic orientation to be made. The technique consists of the patient sitting facing the examiner, who has him open his mouth and stick out his tongue with the aid of a compress, and place the mirror, which has been heated beforehand, against the posterior wall of the oropharynx, pushing back the uvula. The laryngeal mirror is illuminated by Clar's headlamp. The orientation of the mirror allows the different parts of the pharyngolarynx to be visualised and the patient is asked to say "i" or "é", the epiglottis rises and the structures of the larynx are better appreciated. When the nausea reflex is severe, a local anaesthetic is administered by spraying a liquid anaesthetic (Xylocaine with 5% naphazoline).

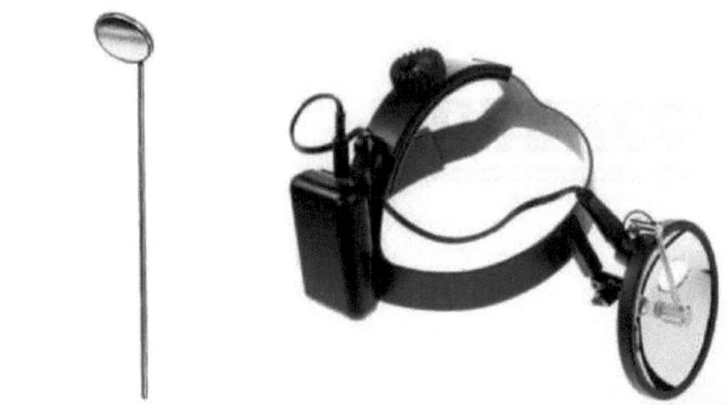

Figure 8: Laryngeal mirror and light source with Clar mirror(34)

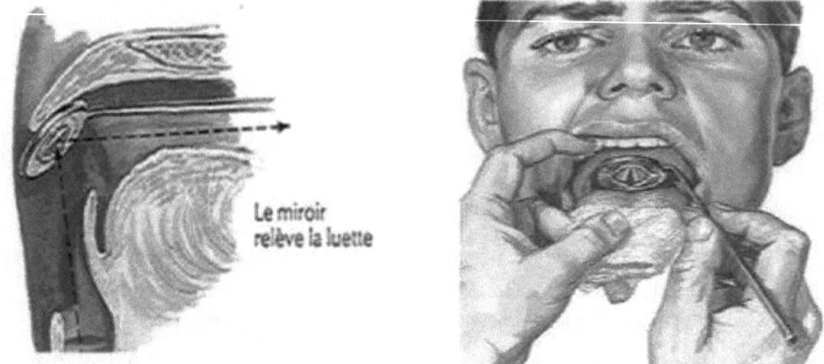

Figure 9: image of the LI(34)

- **Nasofibroscopy:**(32)

The patient sits with an upright torso, leaning slightly forward, with the chin projected slightly upwards and forwards so as to clear the retro-basi-lingual space. The *"sniffing position"* is the equivalent of the Boyce-Jackson position for direct laryngoscopy in suspension: flexion of the neck on the trunk and extension of the head in relation to the cervical spine. Local anaesthesia of the nasal cavities is not systematic. Applying the tip of the fiberscope to the inside of the cheek beforehand limits condensation by depositing saliva. The fiberscope is introduced very gently through the nostril; the patient is asked to ventilate purely through the nose and to relax. The fiberscope is gradually introduced into the nasal cavity and then into the cavum under visual control, in order to be as non-traumatic as possible. As a general rule, the fiberscope should slide over the floor of the nasal cavity, where the nasal passage is widest.

Thanks to nasal ventilation, the soft palate is not contracted. The patient is asked to emit certain phonemes and to swallow. Non-nasal phonemes, such as vowels, are used to study velar contraction. This results in complete occlusion of the nasopharynx, with the soft palate pressing against the posterior nasopharyngeal wall and the soft palate rising. The progression of the nasofibroscope allows observation of the overall morphology of the pharynx and larynx at rest. The mobility of the larynx is studied during phonation, during small expiratory

movements, during coughing efforts (glottic closure) and during sniffing (maximum opening of the glottis) by comparing the two sides.
The mobility of the vocal cord and the arytenoid must be studied separately.

NASOFIBROSCOPE

NASOFIBROSCOPE

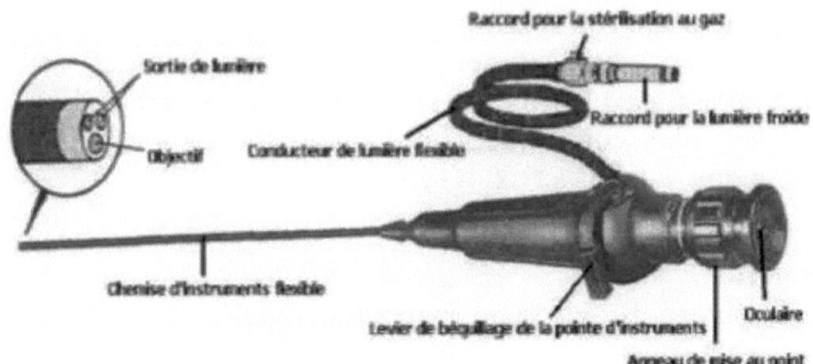

Figure 10: Image of OLYMPUS nasofibroscope(20)

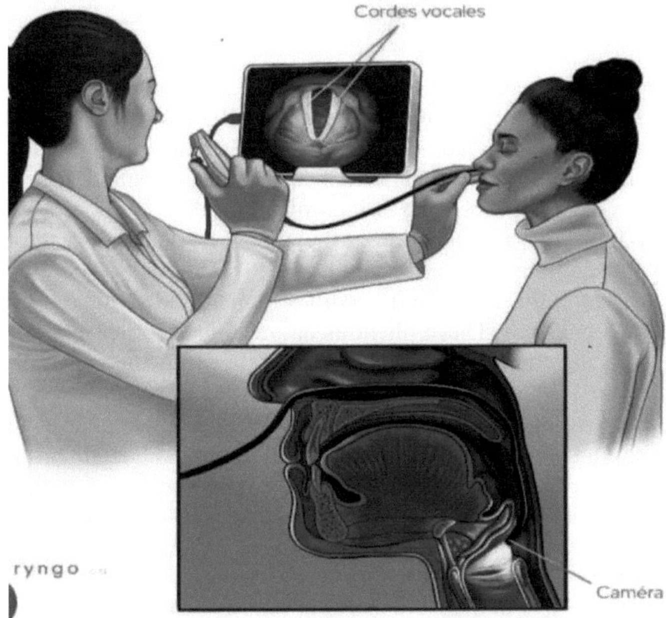

Figure 11: image of a nasofibroscopy (36)

> **Expected outcome of LI and nasofibroscopy:**(30)

In the event of immobility, the arytenoid should be checked for anterior and

medial tilting, atrophy of the cord and its curvature.
The position of the immobile vocal cord must be specified: adducted (medial, phonatory position), paramedian, intermediate (resting) or abducted.
In the case of bilateral involvement, the immobility may be in a paramedian position with the ability to adduct. This is known as glottic dilator paralysis or Gerhardt's syndrome. The paralysis may also be in the adduction position or Riegel's syndrome or, much more rarely, in the abduction position or Ziemssen's syndrome.
In addition to mobility impairment of one or both vocal cords, the extent of associated dysphagia can be assessed by observing salivary stasis in the piriform sinuses and any overflow into the larynx. The cough reflex and laryngeal sensitivity can be assessed by touching the laryngeal margin with the tip of the fiberscope. If the fiberscope passes through to the glottic plane or beyond without any reaction, there is a risk of sensory damage.

> **The different types of RP:** (4,10,22,30)

- **PR Unilateral**

Dysphonia Dysphonia is the main symptom, ranging from hoarseness to a broken voice. There may be a change in timbre with a bitonal voice. High-pitched sounds are difficult to produce. However, dysphonia may be completely absent and the paralysis will only be discovered during laryngoscopy. Swallowing problems are usually absent, but their presence implies damage to the upper laryngeal nerve.
Nasofibroscopy Demonstrates RA: The paralysed vocal cord is usually completely immobile during breathing and when attempting to speak. It usually occupies either a median or paramedian position, or an intermediate position. Complete lateral abduction is exceptional. Occasionally, small movements of the tip of the arytenoid can be seen, which may be related to contraction of the inter-arytenoid muscle or mobilisation of the opposite arytenoid by impact. Over time, the laryngoscopic appearance will change. The arytenoid on the paralysed side tilts forward, and the vocal cord becomes thinner and shorter. It lowers and its edge becomes concave. These phenomena are linked to neurogenic atrophy. The healthy vocal cord sometimes extends beyond the median line to compensate for air leakage. It confronts the paralysed cord when the latter is in the paramedian position. When the paralysis is in the paramedian position, the air leakage is minimal and the voice disorder will quickly be compensated for by the contralateral vocal cord. On the other hand, if the vocal cord is paralysed in the abducted position, the problems will be more serious and will persist longer, due to the hollowness of the glottic cleft.

- **Bilateral PR :**

It is dramatic when it occurs, as it affects not only functional prognosis but also vital prognosis. Bilateral recurrent paralysis is accompanied by more marked disorders, again depending on the position of the vocal cords.

- **Paralysis in closure or adduction**

Dyspnoea is the major feature. It is an inspiratory bradypnoea with supra-sternal and supra-clavicular draught, horniness and turgidity of the jugular veins, often intense and distressing. It can lead to asphyxia if the situation persists, with cyanosis and psychological problems. The patient must then be tracheostomised rapidly. Two elements: whether or not the patient can still speak and indirect laryngoscopy, allow two schematic clinical pictures to be distinguished.

- **Paralysis of the dilators of the glottis or Gerhardt's syndrome:**

Preservation of the voice, which is almost normal, contrasts with the inspiratory bradypnoea which requires numerous breaths to be taken for phonation. Indirect laryngoscopy should be performed with caution in patients at risk of laryngeal spasm. It shows normal vocal cords in a paramedian position. Breathing takes place through a glottic slit of 2 to 3 mm. They do not spread during deep inspiration. They even give the impression of coming together paradoxically, probably as a result of passive inspiration. On the other hand, they clash perfectly during phonation. The characteristic feature of this syndrome is its paroxysmal course. In the context of permanent dyspnoea, attacks of suffocation may occur, giving rise to fears of a life-threatening situation.

- **Global paralysis or Riegel syndrome :**

Inspiratory bradypnoea is associated with dysphonia. The laryngeal organ is completely paralysed in its adduction and abduction movements. It is a complete motor paralysis. This is confirmed by indirect laryngoscopy, which is always dangerous because of the risk of laryngeal spasm. The vocal cords are observed in a paramedian or even median position, completely immobile during both breathing and phonation. It is easy to imagine that the slightest physical effort could lead to respiratory decompensation. The outcome is usually unfavourable.

- **Opening or abduction paralysis or Ziemssen syndrome :**

Aphonia is almost complete. Respiratory problems, which are not asphyxial but are due to a significant flow of air during breathing, indicate a lack of control and regulation of respiratory flow and reflux. They prevent significant or prolonged physical exercise. Indirect laryngoscopy confirms that the glottis is permanently open due to abduction of the vocal cords. The glottic cleft is not modified by respiratory movements or phonation. The glottic gap and the ineffectiveness of tussigenic reflux explain the main danger of this condition: swallowing broncho-pneumopathy. This risk rapidly prohibits the continuation of oral feeding, and may necessitate gastrotomy until laryngeal exclusion can be performed surgically. The outcome can be fatal, due to pulmonary complications.

4.1.2. PARACLINICAL :

Additional diagnostic tests are complex and not commonly performed. The lack of simple objective criteria makes it difficult to determine the frequency of this paralysis.

These include :

> **Single shot:**(30)

In the case of unilateral paralysis, the glottic angle is obliterated, the ventricle and piriform sinus are enlarged, and the paralysed cord is thinned and offset in relation to the healthy cord. In the case of bilateral paralysis, the classic "monkey spanner" image is reversed in the frontal plane due to the enlargement of the ventricles.

> **Stroboscopy:**(3)

This is a key examination in intracordal pathology, used to diagnose and monitor recurrent paralysis when the paralysed vocal cord is sufficiently close to the midline. It is performed in the chair using a 90° lens connected to a stroboscopic light source that emits flashes of light at the desired frequency: by making the frequency of the stroboscope flashes equal to that of the fundamental frequency of the voice, it is possible to examine a larynx at rest and in the different stages of its vibratory cycle by adding a phase difference. This generates a difference between the actual vocal frequency and the illumination frequency. The laryngeal vibration appears asymmetric, slower on the paralysed side in the case of unilateral recurrent damage.

> **Laryngeal electromyography (EMG):**(4,30)

Although it is rarely used in current practice, it is the complementary examination that contributes most to the aetiological diagnosis. It confirms the neurogenic origin of laryngeal immobility, distinguishing between laryngeal paralysis and cricoarytenoid arthritis. It also has prognostic value in monitoring by detecting early signs of regeneration. It is performed under local anaesthetic using a transcutaneous approach: a Bronk needle is inserted into the vocal cord through the cricothyroid membrane. Spontaneous electrical activity at rest or induced by phonation or swallowing is recorded. Nerve conduction velocity is measured after stimulation. This makes it possible to differentiate between nerve sections and simple contusions. This examination must be carried out by a trained operator: it can be a source of undesirable effects which may limit its use in monitoring recovery: pain, vocal cord bleeding, laryngeal spasm, vocal cord oedema, vagal malaise.

> **Types of nerve damage :**

> **According to the Seddon Classification:** (33)

+ Neurapraxia

This is a nerve conduction block with no anatomical damage. The axons are demyelinated, but evoked action potentials are present after supraliminal stimulation. Motor paralysis is complete, with substantial respect for sensory and sympathetic functions. Recovery is complete within variable timescales of up to 12 weeks. The EMG is not alarming, with no fibrillation potential or positive waves.

+ Axonotmesis

This is a loss of axonal continuity, which implies Wallerian degeneration of the distal segment, but the endoneural tubes remain intact. As the endoneurium is not damaged and the basal membrane of the Schwann cells is intact, recovery is generally complete. Only a very proximal lesion, followed by prolonged denervation of the target end organs, will limit functional recovery. Recovery time therefore corresponds to the time taken for axonal regeneration to reach the distal motor targets (average regrowth rate of 1 mm/d). The EMG taken 2 to 3 weeks after nerve damage shows fibrillations and denervation potentials in the musculature downstream of the site.

+ **Neurotmesis**

Neurotmesis is characterised by total sectioning of the nerve or destruction of its internal structure (perineurium and endoneural tubes). There is no action potential, even after stimulation. Fibrillation potentials are characteristic of denervation. Regrowth is associated with axonal misdirection leading to synkinesis. The EMG translation of this lesion is superimposed on that of an axonometric lesion.

> **According to the Sunderland classification:**(34)

+ **First degree nerve damage :**

Is similar to the seddon definition for neurapraxia.

+ **Second degree nerve damage :**

Corresponds to Seddon's definition of axonotmesis.

+ **Third, fourth and fifth degree nerve damage:**

Corresponds to Seddon's neurotmesis.

> **Respiratory function tests:**(30)

It is of little use in extremely urgent situations, where life-saving treatment is required (tracheotomy, intubation) in the face of acute dyspnoea caused by paralysis. In less urgent situations where voice or breathing impairment requires assessment, measurement of maximum flow and analysis of maximum flow-lung volume curves help to define the severity of the obstruction. These measurements are also very useful for assessing therapeutic efficacy.

In the case of variable extra thoracic obstruction such as vocal cord paralysis, the reduction mainly affects inspiratory flow.

> **Voice function measurements:**(10)

Voice assessments consist of a series of examinations, tests, questionnaires and reference scales designed to analyse the voice.

The medical diagnosis is made by a laryngologist or phoniatrist, who examines the state of the ENT sphere: the larynx, vocal cords, resonators, wind tunnel at rest and during phonation, as well as hearing to check the audio phonatory loop in the control of vocal production.

The speech and language therapy assessment complements the medical examination and aims to quantify and qualify the voice using aerodynamic and acoustic measurements, to check how it functions as a gesture, and to record the person's knowledge and beliefs about the voice and their voice. In the event of treatment with medication, surgery or speech therapy, it will form the baseline and will be repeated in order to measure therapeutic effectiveness.

> **Video fluoroscopy:**(30)

It is indicated in cases of dysphagia with or without false routes. It is a useful replacement for the classic swallowing test.

It is used to study laryngeal function during swallowing and the proper coordination of the upper aerodigestive tract.

4.2.DIFFERENTIAL DIAGNOSTCS:(4,30)

- Psychogenic aphonia
- Tumour infiltration (benign, cancer)
- Uni- or bilateral damage to the cricoarytenoid joint (arthritis, ankylosis, dislocation)
- Muscular diseases (myositis, polymyositis, dermatomyositis, muscular dystrophy)

4.3.TREATMENT :

4.3.1. Goals :

4.3.1.1. Unilateral PR :

The challenge is to establish optimal phonation.

4.3.1.2. Bilateral PR :

The aim is to re-establish a sufficient respiratory system without causing swallowing problems.

4.3.2. Resources and instructions :

4.3.2.1. Resources :

4.3.2.1.1. Medical :

> **Corticosteroid therapy :**

If the damage is not known or is not irreversible, during the installation phase, it is useful to give prednisolone at a dose of 1 mg/kg for 5 days by IV followed by decreasing doses per os for 10 days(4,30).

> **Vasodilators, oxygenators, vitamin B :**

They can be proposed (30).

4.3.2.1.2. Speech therapy :

Speech therapy is essential in the treatment of unilateral vocal cord paralysis. It is also useful in bilateral paralysis when vocal quality is impaired (30).

Close observation for 6-12 months is feasible for patients with unilateral VCP with low vocal demands and no risk of aspiration after thyroid surgery. In general, recovery of RA after thyroid surgery occurs within 2-3 months and is less likely to occur after 6-12 months (35).

It is now accepted that speech therapy should be provided early and intensively. Early rehabilitation is an important factor in success, as it helps to minimise maladaptive effort reactions (10).

Exercise programmes include neck extension, laryngeal massage and adjustment of head and neck posture.

Laryngeal massage starts from the surgical site and continues to the surgical site. area in a pain-free range. SLTs educate patients on appropriate posture to reduce muscle tension, in combination with relaxation techniques such as abdominal breathing, yawning, sighing and chewing (36). In severe cases of glottic insufficiency, speech and language therapists may try inhalation and thrust phonation methods (to strengthen the vocal cords). In cases of suspected paralysis of the cricothyroid muscle, gradual shifting up and down the pitch

range (shifting methods) can increase muscle control.
In addition, appropriate global pitch adjustment of speech production subsystems, such as breathing, phonation, resonance and articulation, can reduce excessive stress and improve vocal cord motility and resonant voice quality (37). These techniques include vocal function exercises, the accent method, resonant vocal therapy and semi-occluded vocal tract exercises (38,39). In particular, semi-occluded vocal tract exercises are useful for a variety of organic or behavioural voice disorders, as well as for RA, vocal fatigue and muscle tension dysphonia after thyroid surgery (38).
Vocal abnormalities caused by damage to the recurrent nerve can be considerably improved by voice therapy alone.

4.3.2.1.3. Surgical :

- **Surgical treatment of unilateral RA :**

In unilateral RA, it takes 6 months to intervene, given the possibility of recovery during this period. Surgery is generally performed if speech therapy fails, and uses 2 main procedures to passively medicalise the defective vocal cord:

- **Intracordal injections :**

Various materials can be placed inside the paralysed vocal cord: autologous fat, suspended silicone polymer. These two products are the most widely used in France for this indication. Other materials include autologous fascia and Teflon, the main complication of which is the occurrence of an intracordal foreign body reaction. Bovine collagen does not have marketing authorisation for this indication (40).

- **Thyroplasty**

Thyroplasty consists of placing an inert implant through a window made in the ipsilateral thyroid cartilage wing by cervicotomy. It can be performed under local or loco-regional anaesthetic (40).

- **Other techniques** have been proposed, but remain of limited use: laryngeal adduction, crico-thyroid subluxation and reinnervation.

- **Surgical treatment of bilateral RA :**

Bilateral laryngeal paralysis on closure is the most common.
Treatments therefore usually involve procedures designed to widen the respiratory tract.

- **Tracheotomy**

It is still indicated in cases of acute dyspnoea at the onset of bilateral adduction paralysis, or if the airway is insufficient to tolerate a sedentary lifestyle while waiting for spontaneous recovery. It has the advantage of not making the voice worse. It may even be permanent in patients who do not want any other solution, or in those who do not fit into the indications for reinnervation because of arytenoid fixation and who absolutely want to preserve their voice. If the need for air is not too great, it can be worn with an obturator that will be removed in case of effort, during the night or in case of airway infection (30).

- **Endoscopic removal by CO_2 laser :**

Several techniques are described in the literature, but the 2 main ones are :

- **Posterior segmental cordectomies using the CO_2 laser:**

The technique consists of using a CO_2 laser to cut the vocal cord perpendicularly in its posterior part, through the entire thickness of the thyro-arytenoid muscle. It is performed in front of the vocal apophysis. Depending on the author, the technique may involve a simple posterior cordotomy or a limited resection of the vocal cord (posterior cordectomy) (17).

- **CO_2 laser arytenoidectomy :**

The technique involves removing as much of the arytenoid cartilage as possible without vaporisation. To avoid granuloma formation and denudation of the cricoid, the mucosa covering the arytenoid is preserved (17).

- **Cordopexy :**

The procedure consists of fixing the cord in abduction by simple traction outside or after arytenoidectomy. This method gives good respiratory results. However, the vocal results are poor. This method is generally rarely used (4).

- **Cordectomy :**

A musculoligamentous cordectomy is carried out, extending to the back of the ventricle. The resection is wedge-shaped. It is carried to the limit of the thyroid cartilage. The anterior commissure and vocal process of the arytenoid are respected. It does not alter the flexibility of the hemi-larynx. Cordectomy is unilateral. Several sessions may be necessary (4).

This operation is not associated with haemorrhagic complications. Phonatory results appear to be satisfactory.

There are five types of cordectomy:

Type I: subepithelial cordectomy

Type II: sub-ligament cordectomy

Type III: Trans-muscular cordectomy

Type IV: total cordectomy

Type V: extended cordectomy :

- To the contralateral chord.
- To the arytenoid.
- To the ventricular band.
- Under the glottis.

- **Posterior cordotomy :**

According to Mérite Drancy's method and Laccour's eye.

Using suspension laryngoscopy. Exposure of the

The glottic region shows laryngeal immobility during closure.

Creation of a bilateral "C" notch, measuring laterally around the

4 mm and 2 mm in front of the vocal process of the arytenoids.

The C-shaped notch is located on the posterior 1/3 of both vocal cords in relation to the arytenoids and the preceding 2/3 of the vocal cords. The base of the notch corresponds to the free edge of the vocal cord. Xylocaine with 5% naphazoline on the notched area allows haemostasis to be achieved (2).

- **Total endoscopic arytenoidectomy:**(22)

Ossoff recommends tracheostomy for this type of surgery, which we do not perform systematically.

The larynx can be exposed using a posterior commissure laryngoscope (Ossoff type)

We use a conventional Bouchayer-type laryngoscope, positioned to expose one arytenoid cartilage, the posterior commissure, the inter-arytenoid cleft and at least half of the other arytenoid cartilage. To do this, the 5 or 5.5 mm rubber endotracheal tube is loaded through the laryngoscope and pushed forward. This frees up the operating field and gives a clear view of the arytenoid to be operated on.

- **Partial endoscopic arytenoidectomy:** (4,22)

Includes 2 types:

- **Medial arytenoidectomy :**

The indication applies to cases of less severe dyspnoea and therefore to patients who have not been tracheostomised. This procedure is supposed to reduce the phonatory impact of arytenoidectomy.

The principle is to selectively widen the respiratory glottis without modifying the phonatory glottis or the musculoligamentous insertions of the vocal cords. After vaporisation of the arytenoid muco-perichondrium, the resection is carried out between the vocal process at the front and the postero-medial angle of the arytenoid cartilage at the back. The resection is semicircular and concave medially, 1 to 2 mm deep. The operating time is short. A contralateral procedure may be performed 3 months later if the respiratory result is unsatisfactory.

However, the long-term functional effects on large series of patients have not been documented. Finally, partial arytenoidectomy after cervical radiotherapy is not recommended because of the risk of arytenoid chondro necrosis.

- **Subtotal arytenoidectomy :**

Because of the risk of permanent false routes in the case of total arytenoidectomy, Remacle recommends preserving the pharyngeal side of the arytenoid cartilage.

Removal begins with section of the vocal cord flush with the vocal process and continues laterally and posteriorly into the ventricular floor until it reaches the lateral surface of the arytenoid cartilage.

The section passes through the laryngeal side of the arytenoid cartilage, leaving a pharyngeal side of 2 to 3 mm. The posterior commissure is spared, usually protected by the tracheal intubation tube. Section of the body of the arytenoid cartilage leaves a 2 mm posterior wall and spares the muscular process. The procedure takes between 25 and 30 minutes.

Posterior synechiae may occur. Fluid misdirections are common during the first few days postoperatively and are rapidly compensated for.

- **Cervical surgery**

Several types of procedure have been described. They act on the arytenoid and vocal cord or on the cricoid process to widen the glottic inlet. Other procedures attempt to restore the dilatory function of the glottis by nerve anastomosis or laryngeal neutronisation using a muscle flap with a nerve pedicle (41).

- **Arytenoidopexy or King's operation:**

The principle is to free the muscular and ligamentous attachments of the arytenoid, excluding the vocal muscle, followed by fixation of the arytenoid to the posterior edge of the thyroid wing (41).

- **Arytenoidectomy with cordopexy:** includes,
- **Kelly's Trans thyroidectomy:** (22)

This technique allows arytenoidectomy and pexy of the membranous vocal cord via the Trans thyroidal route. It is not widely used at present, apart from certain teams who reserve it for paediatric cases. The larynx is opened by median thyrotomy. The anterior surface of the arytenoid is incised and the vocal process sectioned. Dissection is performed from front to back, following the cartilage, which must be handled with care because of its fragility. Section of the muscular insertions of the cricoarytenoids, lateral and especially posterior, allows the cartilage to be mobilised. The arytenoid is extracted after sectioning the cricoarytenoid joint.

- **Retro-arytenoid arytenoidectomy or Graâf-Woodnan procedure:**(4)

Unlike King's technique, Woodman resects the body of the arytenoid cartilage and performs a pexy of the vocal process on the small horn of the thyroid cartilage. This technique should be used if the arytenoid ruptures during an arytenoidopexy.

- **Speech by Rethi :**

This involves performing a partial or total thyrotomy and sectioning the cricoid neck. The gap is maintained either by a cartilaginous material or by a dilating prosthesis, until fibrous tissue fills the posterior inter-cricoid space (41).

- **Reinnervation techniques:**(25)

Whereas Crumley's technique of anastomosis of the descending branch of the XII to the adductor branch of the recurrent appears to be sufficient on its own in cases of paralysis of the adductors, Tucker's technique of reinnervation of the lateral cricothyroid muscle via the omohyoid musculo-nervous pedicle should ideally be combined with thyroplasty. Various authors have been able to reproduce Crumley's results. Marie combines reinnervation with fat injection to provide a temporary solution.

The results of these techniques remain disappointing.

- **Laryngeal pacemaker for swallowing disorders :**

This procedure is currently being tested.

However, laboratory and clinical trials have been carried out by Broniatowski with the aim of re-establishing coordinated and dynamic swallowing by directly stimulating the recurrent nerve or the vagus nerve, or by creating a reflex arc between a skin flap implanted in the pharynx and having retained its sensitive innervation and the recurrent nerve(30).

- **Suture of the epiglottis to the laryngeal margin:** (4)

In 1972 Habbal and Murray proposed suturing the epiglottis to the laryngeal margin by pharyngotomy. The edges of the laryngeal margin and epiglottis are incised and dissected, and the suture is made in two planes.

- **Suturing the vocal cords together:**(22)

In 1975, Montgomery proposed that the vocal cords be opened and sutured together by thyrotomy. Kitahara also proposed suturing the ventricular bands, while Sasaki covered the suture with a flap of sternohyoid muscle with a superior pedicle sutured to the posterior commissure.

- **Tracheoesophageal diversion:**(30)

Lindemann in 1975 and Krespi in 1984 proposed separating the trachea from the larynx by sectioning the trachea at the level of the third ring. The trachea is anastomosed to the skin, while the larynx is anastomosed to the oesophagus. The disadvantage of this technique is the accumulation of saliva at the back of the larynx, which tends to encourage diverticulum. The technique is potentially reversible.

- **Plicature of the epiglottis:**(30)

In 1983, Biller proposed a vertical supraglottic closure by tubulating the epiglottis. However, an upper orifice remains, which also facilitates saliva inhalation.

- Total laryngectomy :

Effective but mutilating, total laryngectomy is a possibility to be considered for the permanently impotent patient (41).

4.3.2.2 Indications :

Management of RA involves corticosteroid-based treatment to reduce the inflammation and laryngeal oedema that can cause symptoms to worsen.

However, studies have shown that systemic administration of corticosteroids is not recommended to improve voice quality after thyroid surgery (35).

- **Unilateral PR :**

Voice therapy can be used to improve vocal outcomes in patients with mild symptoms or if surgical mediation procedures are not available (42).

In the absence of life-threatening swallowing disorders, speech therapy is the first-line treatment option. Surgery is indicated:

- rapidly in cases of severe dysphonia or threatening swallowing disorders - when the functional result achieved by rehabilitation appears insufficient. Scientific data do not allow us to set a time limit, which must be discussed on an individual basis (40).

- **Bilateral PR :**
- **Closing:**

The challenge in this case is to restore breathing as quickly as possible, based on 2 principles:

- Tracheotomy, which preserves the anatomy of the larynx, performed immediately in an emergency.
- Endoscopic techniques that avoid or attempt to eliminate the need for tracheostomy.

The choice will depend on a number of factors to be taken into consideration: the certainty or otherwise of nerve section, the definitive nature of the paralysis, the inflammatory aspect of the larynx, the post-intubation context, the patient's wishes as expressed pre-operatively, the patient's age and general condition, the local conditions of the centres (laser equipment), and the experience of the operator (40).

Arytenoidectomy with or without cordopexy usually gives excellent results (41). This operation should not be delayed too long, as crico-arytenoid ankylosis is inevitable after a certain time, especially if the patient has been intubated and ventilated for more than 5 or 6 days before the tracheotomy.

- **Opening ceremony:**

Bilateral opening paralysis, or Ziemsen's syndrome, is certainly exceptional but has a very poor prognosis and is extremely difficult to treat(22); there are vital risks due to the extent of false routes.

Depending on the severity of the swallowing problems and the risk of pulmonary infections, adapting food textures, stopping oral feeding, performing a gastrostomy or a cuffed tracheostomy are only options in the interim, given the risks of inhalation(4,40).

Laryngeal exclusion is a possibility to be considered in the permanently impotent patient (4).

4.3.3. Evolution :

Recurrent paralysis may be transient or permanent. Some authors consider that RA is permanent after 6 months(43). Others do not consider RA to be permanent until after 12 months (43,44).

In general, recovery from vocal cord paralysis after thyroid surgery occurs within 2-3 months and is less likely to occur after 6-12 months (35).

In bilateral recurrent paralysis, the prognosis can be life-threatening if not treated urgently (4).

4.3.4. Prevention :

Prevention of RA is both preoperative and intraoperative.

A search for pre-existing laryngeal damage is recommended if the initial clinical examination reveals dysphonia or if there is a history of cervicotomy (45).

Intraoperatively, prevention requires careful dissection, avoidance of excessive traction, and judicious choice of haemostasis techniques and of the approach to the recurrent nerve (46).

In the American recommendations, three methods of visualisation of the inferior laryngeal nerve are recommended: the lateral, inferior or superior approach (24). The lateral approach is the most commonly used for simple thyroidectomies. The thyroid lobe is retracted medially, the middle thyroid vein is individualised and the recurrent nerve is identified at the middle pole. The inferior approach is recommended for revision or goitre surgery. The nerve is located in the tracheo-oesophageal sulcus, where it crosses the ATI. With the superior approach, the recurrent nerve is identified at its crossing point under the inferior pharyngeal constrictor muscle, close to the cricothyroid junction (47,48). Non-recurrence of the inferior laryngeal nerve is an anatomical variant that the surgeon should be aware of. It always occurs on the right and is associated with an absence of the brachiocephalic arterial trunk and retrooesophageal passage of the subclavian

artery (arteria lusoria).
To help the surgeon identify it, intra-operative neuro-stimulation of the inferior laryngeal nerve has been proposed as likely to reduce the risk of recurrent paralysis(25).
As far as haemostasis techniques are concerned, the classic methods - ligatures, application of clips, monopolar or bipolar haemostasis, which is more elective - and the new means of haemostasis - thermofusion and the energy produced by ultrasound - are widely used, often in combination, depending on the habits of each surgeon (9,45).

CHAPTER II

METHODOLOGY

1-Setting and place of study

The study was carried out in the Department of Otorhinolaryngology and Cervicofacial Surgery at the Gabriel Touré University Hospital in Bamako, Mali.

1.1.Presentation of the Gabriel Touré University Hospital

- **History :**

Formerly known as the Bamako Central Dispensary, Gabriel Touré Hospital is one of Bamako's university hospital centres.

It currently has 447 beds and employs 763 staff in all categories, including 181 on contract.

Baptised Gabriel Touré on 7 January 1959, in memory of a young Sudanese man. He was a medical student who died on 12 June 1934 as a result of contamination during a plague epidemic.

He was part of the younger generation of Africa's first doctors.

- **Geographical location :**

Located in commune III of the district of Bamako, the Gabriel Touré University Hospital covers an area of 3 hectares 28 ares 54 centiares. It is bordered to the east by the Médina-Coura district, to the west by the Abderrahmane Baba Touré national engineering school, to the south by the railway estate and to the north by the General Staff of the armed forces and the ministerial reserve squadron.

- **Its infrastructure:** includes :

S General management

S An admissions office with various outpatient cubicles.

S A Department of Medicine, including Gastroenterology, Neurology, Cardiology and Diabetology.

S A paediatrics department with general paediatrics, neonatology and oncology services.

J A medical-technical department comprising the medical imaging department and the functional exploration department.

J A hospital pharmacy department.

J A surgery department :

- General surgery ;
- Paediatric surgery ;
- Otolaryngology and cervicofacial surgery (ENT and CCF) ;
- Traumatology and orthopaedics ;
- Neurosurgery ;
- Urology ;
- Physical medicine (physiotherapy).

J A medical biology department comprising the biomedical analysis laboratory and the blood transfusion service.

J A department of anaesthesia-intensive care and emergency medicine :
- Emergency department (SAU) ;
- Adult resuscitation ;
- Medical regulation ;
- Anaesthesia ;
- Operating theatre.

J A gynaecology-obstetrics department :
- Gynaecology ;
- Obstetrics ;
- Two operating theatres.

Services such as maintenance and social services are staffed at management level.
The hygiene and sanitation unit and the laundry are attached to the general surveillance department, the mortuary to the medical department and the kitchen to the administrative department.
Each department is headed by a department head

I.I.IPresentation of the ENT and CCF department

- **Human resources :**

The ENT department is a medical-surgical department headed by a full professor, assisted by a full professor plus three senior lecturers, three research fellows and two hospital otorhinolaryngologists.
The department has :
S Twenty-three doctors registered for a DES ;
S Eight ENT specialist medical assistants;
S Two senior health technicians ;
S A health technician ;
S An executive secretary ;
S Two surface technicians ;
S A care assistant ;
S Thesis students from the Faculty of Medicine and Odontostomatology in Bamako (FMOS).

- **The infrastructure of the service includes :**

S A consultation unit with :
- Two (02) consultation cubicles
- A functional exploration unit (audio-impedancemetry)
- An inpatient unit: 11 rooms, including 3 VIP inpatient rooms, with a total capacity of 28 beds
- An on-call room for DES and PhD students
- An on-call room for medical assistants
- An on-call room for surface technicians
- Two (02) operating theatres not yet operational and a sterilisation room
- An office for the head of department
- An office for the hospital unit manager
- Five (05) offices for doctors

- A meeting/training room
- A toilet with three (3) WCs and a shower for staff
- A toilet with three (03) WCs and a shower for patients

1.2 Type of study

This was an observational, descriptive study with retrospective recruitment.

1.3 The study period

The study will run for 25 months, from January 2021 to January 2023.

1.4 Sampling

> **Inclusion criteria :**

■ Any patient having consulted for dysphonia, dyspnoea after thyroidectomy.

■ Any patient who has consulted for other laryngeal symptoms following thyroidectomy.

■ With immobility of one or more vocal cords on nasofibroscopy or suspension laryngoscopy.

■ **Non-inclusion criteria** :

■ Survey form incorrectly filled in.

■ Refusal to take part in the study.

■ Cases of post-thyroidectomy cricoarytenoid arthritis or dislocation

1.5 Data collection technique

The information was obtained using our questionnaire drawn up for this purpose, or by the patient himself. The data were recorded on our survey form.

1.6 Study variables

■ Socio-epidemiological situation: age, sex, profession, place of residence and antecedents.

■ Clinical data: reason for consultation, history, associated signs, ENT examination, characteristics of pre- and post-thyroidectomy laryngeal signs (mode of onset, types, rhythm and calming and triggering factors), characteristics of thyroid pathology, operator, surgical procedure, state of vocal cords (results of nasofibroscopy), therapeutic management of recurrent paralysis, post-operative follow-up at 3 months, 12 months, etc.

1.7 Computerised data

The data will be entered into SPSS software version 19.0 containing a data entry mask based on a survey form.

1.8 Data processing and analysis

The data were analysed using SPSS

The graphics were produced using EXCEL office 2019.

1.9 How it works

A procedure was used to enrol patients according to the inclusion criteria.

1.10 The ethical aspect

This is a purely scientific study aimed at understanding the epidemiological, diagnostic and therapeutic aspects of post-thyroidectomy recurrent paralysis at Gabriel Toure University Hospital. The results will be used to improve the quality of care. The consent of patients or their relatives (accompanying persons) will be obtained beforehand.

CHAPTER III

RESULTS

1. Socio-demographic aspects :

The study lasted 15 months. During this study period, 27 patients were registered.

Figure 1: Breakdown of patients by age

Age range	Frequency	Percentage
[20 to 30 years [	4	14,8
[31 to 40 years old [	4	14,8
[41 to 50 years [	**12**	**44,4**
[51 to 60 years [	2	7,5
[61 to 70 years old [	5	18,5
Total	27	100,0

The most represented age group was **41 to 50**, or **44.4%, with extremes ranging from** 23 **to 70**, and an average **age** of **46.18**.

■ **Sex**

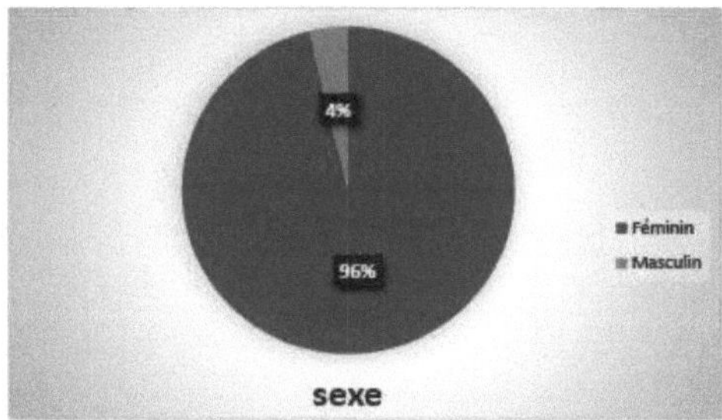

Figure 12: Breakdown of patients by gender.

Females accounted for 96%**.** The sex ratio was 0.04.

■ **Profession**

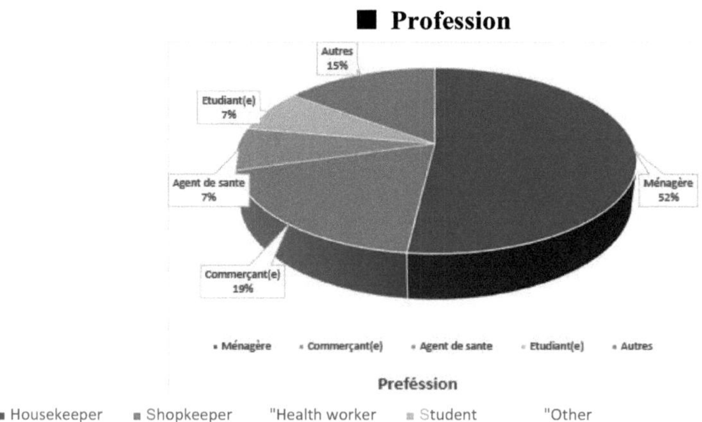

Preference

Other: teacher and restorer.

Figure 13: Breakdown of patients by profession.

Housewives were the most represented at **52%.**

Table II: Breakdown of patients by mode of recruitment

Recruitment method	Frequency	Percentage
Consultation box	**24**	**88,9**
Emergency department	3	11,1
Total	27	100,0

The majority of our patients (**88.9%**) were enrolled in the **consultation cubicles**.

2. Diagnostic aspects

2.1.Contributing factors:

■ On histology, in all our patients the **tumour was benign**, i.e. **100%** of cases.

Tableau III: Distribution of patients according to indication for thyroidectomy

Indications for thyroidectomy	Frequency	Percentage
Basedow's disease	**14**	**51,9**
Multi-nodular goitre	11	40 ,7
Plunging goitre	2	7,4
Total	27	100,0

Basedow disease was the main indication for surgery, with 14 cases (**51.9%**).

Tableau IV: Breakdown of patients by type of thyroidectomy

Surgical procedure	Frequency	Percentage
Total thyroidectomy	**20**	**74,1**
Subtotal thyroidectomy	3	11,1
Left lobo-isthmectomy	3	11,1
Right lobo-isthmectomy	1	3,7
Total	27	100,0

Total thyroidectomy was performed in 20 cases (**74.1%**).

All our patients were operated on by general surgeons.

Tableau V: Breakdown of patients by recurrence search

Recurrent search	Frequency	Percentage
Unknown	17	63
Not carried out	5	18,5
Made with lesions	**5**	**18,5**
Total	27	100,0

No information was given on recurrent search in 63% of cases.

2.2 Clinical signs

Table VI: Breakdown of patients according to post-Th

Clinical manifestations	Frequency	Percentage

Dyspnoea+Dysphonia	22	81,5
Isolated dysphonia	4	14,8
Isolated dyspnoea	1	3 ,7
Dysphagia	6	22,2
Dry cough	4	14,8
Hypersialorrhea	4	14,8

Dyspnoea and dysphonia were associated in **81.5%** of cases and isolated in **3.7%** and **14.8%** respectively.
Dysphagia was the third major sign in 22.**2%** of patients.

2.2.1. characteristics of dyspnoea

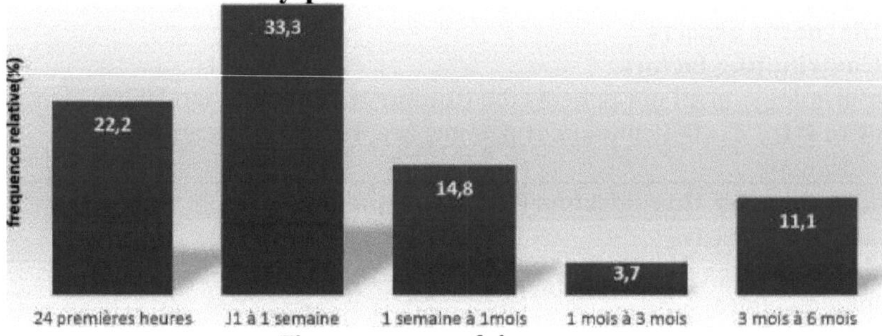

Figure 14: Distribution of patients according to time to onset of dyspnoea

Dyspnoea appeared in the first 24 hours **22.2% after thyroidectomy and** in **the first week** in **33.3%.**

Table VII: Distribution of patients according to dyspnoea staging according to Chevalier Jackson and Pineau

Jackson and Pineau knight classification	Frequency	Percentage
Stage I	2	7,4
Stage II	1	3,7
Stage III	**20**	**74,1**
Stage IV	00	00
Total	23	85,2

Inspiratory dyspnoea was classified as **stage III** in **74.1%** of patients.

2.2.2. Characteristics of dysphonia :

Table VIII: Distribution of patients according to voice quality

Voice quality	Frequency	Percentage
Voices	**16**	**59,3**
Rauque		
Bitonal voice	8	29,6
Tired voice	2	7,4

Total	26	96 ,3

The voice was **hoarse** in **59.3%** of cases.

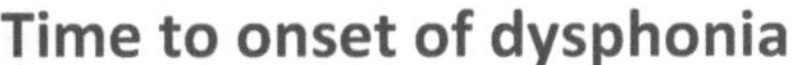

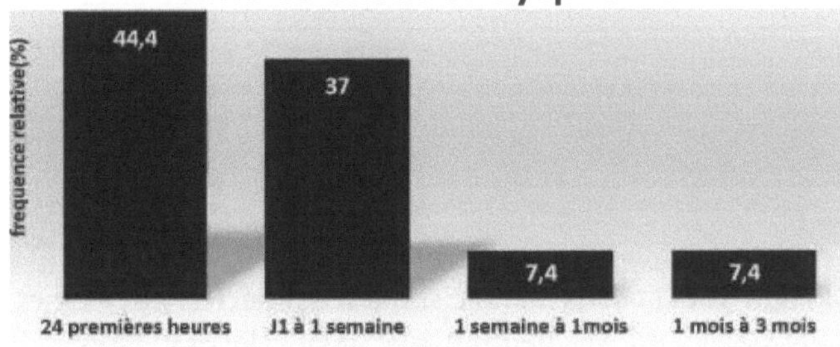

Figure 15: Distribution of patients according to time to onset of dysphonia

Dysphonia appeared within the first 24 hours after thyroidectomy in 12 cases **(44.4%).**

2.2.3. Nasofibroscope examination :

Table IX: Breakdown of patients by type of recurrent paralysis

Types	Frequency	Percentage
Laryngeal diplegia (Bilateral)	**21**	**77,8**
Monoplegia (Unilateral)	6	22,2
Total	27	100,0

Laryngeal diplegia accounted for **77.8% of cases.**

2.2.3.1. Characteristics of diplegia :

Table X: Distribution of patients according to vocal cord and arytenoid characteristics in diplegic disorders

Nasofibroscopy of laryngeal diplegia	Workforce	Percentage
Vocal strings		
-Supply	21	100
-Paramedian	21	100
-Atrophied	17	80,9
-Incurved	**04**	**19,1**
Arytenoids		
-Bilateral fixity	21	100
-Tilted forward	21	100

The vocal cords were in the **paramedian position** in **100%** of cases.
The vocal cords were atrophic in **80.9%** and curved in 19.1%.
The **arytenoids were fixed and tilted** forward in **100%** of cases.

2.2.3.2. Characteristics of laryngeal monoplegia :

Table XI: Distribution of patients according to the characteristics of the vocal cord and arytenoid affected in monoplegia

Laryngeal monoplegia nasofibroscopy	Right vocal chord		Left vocal chord	
	Frequencies	Percentage	Frequencies	Percentage
Vocal cord				
-median	3	50%	3	50%
-fix	3	50%	3	50%
Arytenoids				
-fix	3	50%	3	50%
-tilted forward	3	50%	3	50%

The **left and right vocal cords** had the **same frequencies**, i.e. **3 cases** each. In all cases, the vocal cord was **median and fixed (100%** of cases).
The arytenoid on the affected side was **fixed and tilted forward** in **100%** of cases.

3 Therapeutic aspects :

Table XII: Breakdown of patients according to the time taken for treatment after thyroidectomy

Delay	Frequency	Percentage
Less than 24 hours	1	3,7
D1 to one week	**17**	**63**
1 to 3 months	5	18,5
3 to 6 months	1	3,7
6 to 12 months	2	7,4
More than 12 months	1	3,7
Total	27	100,0

Approximately **63%** of our patients were managed within the first six months.

Table XIII: Breakdown of patients by therapeutic method

Therapeutic means	Frequency	Percentage
Methylprednisolone	27	100,0
Speech therapy	**21**	**77,8**
Tracheotomy	20	74,1
Post-transverse cordotomy	20	74,1

All our patients received **intravenous** corticosteroid therapy with **methylprednisolone (1mg/kg)** for **5 days** and **oral corticosteroid** therapy for **10 days. Speech therapy** was used in the majority of cases (**77.8%**).
Tracheostomy was performed in 20 cases, i.e. **74.1%** of cases.
Posterior cordotomy was the surgical treatment, with 20 patients (**74.1%**) benefiting from this procedure.
NB: all cordotomies were performed using endoscopic micro forceps.

Table XIV: Breakdown of time taken to complete speech therapy treatment

Deadline	Frequency	Percentage
Less than 2 months	5	23,8

2 to 3 months	**16**	**76,2**
Total	21	100

The time taken to complete speech therapy was **2 to 3 months (76.2%).**

Table XV: Distribution of patients according to the time required for transverse posterior cordotomy using endoscopic micro forceps

Deadlines	Frequency	Percentage
One week after thyroidectomy	4	20
6 to 12 months	16	**80**
Total	20	100

Posterior cordotomy was performed **6 to 12 months after corticotherapy** in 16 cases, i.e. **80%.**

■ **Haemorrhage** was the intraoperative complication in **100%** of cases. This haemorrhage was controlled by applying xylocaine with 5% naphazoline to the notch.

3. Evolution :

Table XVI: Distribution of patients according to the state of the glottic tract after posterior transverse cordotomy

> **Bilateral RP**

Status of the glottic tract	Délaide		Monitoring	
	3 months	6 months	9 months	12 months
Good	18(90%)	18(90%)	18(90%)	20(100%)
Bad	2(10%)	2(10%)	2(10%)	00
		1ère trade-in	2ème trade-in	

At 3ème , 6ème , 9ème months:

A follow-up nasofibroscopy was performed after the posterior transverse cordotomy, which revealed a good glottic airway in **90%** of cases. In 10% of cases, the glottic airway was insufficient in some patients.

At 12ème months, good vocal cord mobility was observed in all patients.

■ The **mortality** rate was **3.7%.**

> **Unilateral RA**

From 3ème to 12ème months, good vocal cord mobility was observed at nasofibroscopy in all monoplegic patients.

CHAPTER IV

COMMENTS AND DISCUSSION

1 Methodological aspects :

1.1.Difficulties encountered :

Our study was conducted in the Otorhinolaryngology and Cervicofacial Surgery Department of the Gabriel Touré University Hospital. Its aim was to study the epidemiological, diagnostic and therapeutic aspects of RA.

During the course of our work, we encountered a number of difficulties in producing our results:

- Non-compliance with treatment
- The non-availability and defective quality of certain materials: Nasofibroscopy and transverse posterior cordotomy equipment
- The approach to the recurrent nerve in the thyroid cavity is often unclear.
- The absence of recurrent nerve monitoring in our context

2 . Epidemiological aspect :

2.1.Frequency :

Recurrent paralysis (RP) is the most common and feared complication of thyroid surgery (3).

This complication has been described since the early days of thyroid surgery, with a rate of 32% in 1844 for Bill Roth (44).

The incidence of recurrent inferior laryngeal nerve complications in African and international literature is currently between 2 and 6% (5).

According to a study published by **Hung Chun Chen et all** , the incidence of vocal cord paralysis caused by thyroid surgery ranges from 1.5% to 5.3% (6).

CL KONESSA et all reported an incidence of recurrent paralysis of 3.8% in 155 thyroidectomies performed over 3 years (49).

In a study carried out in Mali by **T. Sissoko et all**, recurrent lesions accounted for 2.8% of complications in 158 thyroidectomies performed over a period of 5 years (9).

According to **Rosato et all**, the percentage of bilateral recurrent paralysis is 0.4% (7). This paralysis would be permanent in 1 to 3% of surgeries and temporary in 5 to 8% (50).

We recorded 27 cases of recurrent paralysis over a period of 3 years, giving an annual frequency of 9 cases per year.

2.2.Age

The age of patients with RA ranged from 23 to 70 years, with an average of **46.18 years**. In our study, **44.4% of** patients were between **41 and 55 years of** age. Our data are consistent with those of **Lamia Dbab et all and Wafea Zarari et all**, who found the age range most represented to be 40 to 49 years and 33 to 56 years respectively (3.22). This could be explained by the fact that, generally speaking, the average age of thyroid pathology varies between 40 and 60, and is therefore the preserve of young adults (51,52).

2.3.Gender :

The predominance of women in our study is comparable to that of **Lamia Dbad**

et all and **Renata Mizusaki et all** who respectively had **83%** with a sex ratio of 0.2 and **86.1%, i.e. a sex ratio** of 0.16 in favour of women (3.53). This female predominance has been described by many other authors and could be justified by the high incidence of thyroid disease in women, which bears witness to the role played by the presence of sex steroid receptors in the follicular cells of the thyroid (44,54).

2.4.Recruitment method :

The majority of our patients (**88.9%**) were admitted to the consulting room and **11.1%** to the emergency department.

3 Clinical and anatomopathological aspects :

3.1.Contributing factor :

3.1.1. Clinical :

Prevention of RA is both preoperative and intraoperative. Preoperatively, if the initial clinical examination reveals dysphonia or if there is a history of cervicotomy, a systematic pre- and postoperative laryngoscopy should be performed to check for pre-existing laryngeal damage (9,45).

In our study, our patients did not undergo preoperative laryngoscopy and none had laryngeal symptoms prior to thyroidectomy.

3.1.2. Histological types :

The anatomopathological results of the surgical specimens showed no signs of malignancy in any of our patients, i.e. **100%** benign cases. **Lamia Dbad et all** found benign cases in 91.6% (3).

The absence of thyroid cancer cases in our study is explained by the size of our sample. Thyroid cancer is the main factor favouring RA due to nerve infiltration.

3.1.3. Indication for thyroidectomy :

Graves' disease was the main indication for surgery in **51.9%** of cases, followed by multinodular goitres in **40.7%.** Our results are similar to those of **CL KONESSA et all** whose 33% of indications were Basedow disease and multinodular goitres (49). The surgical indications are diverse, the isolated nodule and the basedowified goitre were found in 25% in the series of Lamia Dbab et all (3). Multi-nodular goitre and compressive goitre were the surgical indications in other series (22).

The high rate of PR after thyroidectomy for Graves' disease is linked to the technical difficulties recognised by the operators due to chronic inflammation and increased local vascularisation, which would increase complications (55). Graves' disease presents certain particularities in relation to thyroid surgery: any kind of pathology confused with an enlarged gland exerts a compressive effect on the recurrent nerves, which are laminated posteriorly, making them difficult to dissect and explaining the possibility of recurrent paralysis (4,22,44).

On the other hand, a study by **Roulet Maxim et all** and by **A. Beit et all** and many other authors concluded that there was no significant difference in the occurrence of recurrent paralysis and the other usual complications associated with thyroidectomy between patients operated on for Graves' disease and others (56,57).

3.1.4. Type of thyroidectomy :

In our study, the most common surgical procedure was total thyroidectomy (**74.1%**). Our results are similar to those of **Renata Mizusaki et all** (53) who found **88%** of total thyroidectomy. This could be explained by the fact that, as total thyroidectomy is nothing other than a duplicate of lobectomy, the risk of recurrence is multiplied by two, as both nerves are exposed. In advanced neoplastic disease, total thyroidectomy is often associated with unilateral or bilateral central lymph node dissection and possibly resection of the surrounding muscles; the nerve is exposed to section, stretching or sacrifice out of necessity (22). The risk of RA is present whatever the thyroid procedure. The type of surgery (re-operation), the underlying thyroplasty, the extent of resection and the volume of activity of the surgeon are all involved (45).

3.1.5. Intraoperative recurrence search :

In our sample, we had no information on nerve dissection in **63% of** cases, dissection was not performed in **18.5% of** cases, and the lesion was confirmed in **18.5%** of cases, including one case of stretching and 4 cases of accidental section of the recurrent nerve.

Intraoperatively, the prevention of RA involves the identification and systematic dissection of the recurrent laryngeal nerve (44,45).

There are three possible approaches to the recurrent nerve, each with its own advantages and disadvantages. The lateral approach is the most commonly used. In the event of a repeat operation, the inferior approach is safer, and when the goitre is large, the superior approach is preferable. In all cases, identification of the recurrent must be systematic (9,24).

Other factors have been suggested:The nerve entangled in a fibrous mesh of Berry ligament, the relationship of the nerve with ATI(pre-vascular and trans-vascular), the non-recurrent nerve, haemostasis with an electric scalpel less than one millimetre from the nerve, the number of dividing branches of the recurrent, the anterior branches always being motor, the thinnest nerves appearing to be the most fragile, the size of the recurrent, cervical hyperextension (which stretches the nerve) (47,48,58).

In recent decades, several technologies have been used for nerve monitoring to prevent damage to the recurrent laryngeal nerve (59).

In our study, all patients were operated on by general surgeons and none by ENT surgeons. The systematic absence of recurrent research associated with these factors would be responsible for the increased rate of recurrent morbidity in our study. Knowledge of the anatomy and anatomical variations of the recurrent nerve and the surgeon's experience reduce the risk of recurrent paralysis.

3.2.Diagnostic aspect :

3.2.1. Clinical :

In our study inspiratory dyspnoea and dysphonia were associated in **81.5%**, dysphonia was isolated in **14.8%** and dyspnoea in **3.7%**. **Lamia Dbad et all** found dysphonia to be the main functional sign (3).

In our study, the onset of dyspnoea was within the first 24 hours in **22.2%**, within the first week after thyroidectomy in **33.3%**, one week to 1 month in 14.8%, 1 to 3 months in 3.7%, 3 to 6 months in 11.1%; according to the Chevalier Jackson and Pineau classification, dyspnoea was classified as **stage III** in **74.1%.**

Dysphonia had set in within the first 24 hours in **44.4%** of cases, within the first week in 37%, within the first month in 7.4%, between 1 and 3 months in 7.4%, and was **hoarse** in **59.3%** of cases.

Swallowing disorders of the fossa route type were present in **22.2%**; dry cough and hypersialorrhoea in **14.8%**.

Our data are consistent with the literature, which describes swallowing difficulties and coughing as the main associated signs (10).

This could be explained by damage to the external branch of the superior laryngeal nerve or by glottic incompetence resulting from vocal cord paresis or paralysis. This reduces the ability to develop subglottic pressure for effective swallowing (10).

Stroboscopy and electromyography are essential for making a positive diagnosis of neurogenic damage to the recurrent nerves. As these examinations were not accessible in our context, nasofibroscopy enabled us to describe the various lesions. It was performed systematically on all patients. Laryngeal diplegia accounted for **77.8%**. They are rare and difficult to quantify in the literature, around 0.4% according to **Rosato et all** (7).

The 2 vocal cords were **fixed and paramedian in 100% of cases of diplegia**, **atrophied** in **80.9%** and curved in **19.1%**, and the 2 arytenoids were **fixed** and **tilted forward** in all cases.

The high frequency of diplegia in our study could be explained by the high frequency of total thyroidectomy in our study, which increases the risk of injury to the 2 recurrent nerves.

In monoplegia, the left and right vocal cords were affected at the same frequency in 3 cases each, i.e. 22.2%. They were **fixed and medial** with the arytenoid of the affected side **tilted forward** in all cases. This result differs from that of **Lamia Dbad et all** who found 1.2% of unilateral RA.

3)).

In the literature, right-sided RA is more common than left-sided RA, as on the right side the recurrent nerve is located anterior to the inferior thyroid artery and on the lateral aspect of the trachea, whereas on the left side the nerve is retroarterial and is found in the oesotracheal dihedral angle (4).

The fact that both vocal cords were equally affected may be explained by the size of our sample.

4) Therapeutic aspect :

4.1.Duration of treatment :

In our study, **63% of** our patients were managed within the first week after thyroidectomy, including cases of diplegia and monoplegia. This delay in treatment is related to the delay in aggravation of symptoms such as inspiratory dyspnoea and dysphonia.

1.2 Monoplegia :

The management of monoplegia is well codified, and speech therapy is the first-line treatment(1,10). It was systematically applied to all our patients. We opted for medical treatment with methylprednisolone. According to **Hwan Ryu et all**, voice therapy is useful for improving voice quality and quality of life in patients with voice problems after thyroid surgery (35). In general, recovery from vocal cord paralysis after thyroid surgery occurs within 2-3 months and is less likely to occur after **6-12 months.** In our study, speech rehabilitation was systematic in **100%** of cases of monoplegia; in the majority of cases it took 2 to 3 months after thyroidectomy.

If medical treatment fails within 6-12 months of follow-up, surgery such as vocal cord medialization may be performed. In the literature, the incidence of transient RA varies between **1.4%** and **38.4%** (50).

1.3. Diplegia :

In our sample, all the cases of diplegia were permanent; some authors consider that RA is permanent after a period of 6 months (43), while others consider that RA is definitive only after a period of 12 months (44). Our study does not agree with that of **J-P. Jeannon et all**, who found, after a review of the literature, an incidence of permanent RA of between **0% and 18.6%** (50).

This difference may be explained by the fact that some surgeons do not systematically locate and dissect the recurrent nerve in our context, which could reduce the risk of irreversible damage to the recurrent nerve. In our sample, tracheostomy was performed to improve dyspnoea in 20 patients **(74.1%).** This could be explained by the fact that in our study the number of patients with diplegia was dyspnoeic, classified as stage III by Chevalier Jackson and Pineau. Transverse partial posterior cordotomy is the gold standard treatment. It is quick and easy to perform, and limits swallowing problems, preserves good phonation and has no serious complications, making it the method of choice in the first instance. If it fails, it can be repeated and/or performed bilaterally(8). We performed it in **74.1% of** cases. There was one case of death before posterior cordotomy **(3.7%).** The time taken to perform a transverse posterior cordotomy depends on the functional recovery of the nerve, with a waiting period of 6-12 months. In better-equipped centres, this delay is reduced thanks to data from laryngeal electromyography and stroboscopy. In our context of a technical picture of deficient work, we based ourselves on the results of the operative report from surgeons affirming the nerve lesion, and the waiting time of 6-12 months in cases where no status of the inferior laryngeal nerve was given intraoperatively. In **80%** of cases, cordotomy was performed within 6 to 12 months in the absence of vocal cord mobility. This therapeutic decision has been reported in the literature, and in 4 patients cordotomy was performed within the first week, in whom intraoperative recurrent nerve section was confirmed.

Posterior cordotomy is a compromise between breathing and phonation, and is not without complications. The main complication was intraoperative haemorrhage. Haemostasis was achieved by applying xylocaine with 5% naphazoline to the raw part of the notch. Intraoperative haemorrhage has been

reported in **11.1%** of cases (2).
After surgery, speech therapy was used in **75%** of cases.

2. Evolution :

Normally, nasofibroscopy was performed in almost all patients who underwent cordotomy **(96.3%)**. One patient died before cordotomy, representing 3.7% of the sample. From 3ème to 9ème months, good vocal cord mobility was observed in all patients with monoplegic impairment corresponding to the transient RA rate. In patients with laryngeal diplegia after transverse posterior cordotomy, a good glottic tract was observed, with a stable "C" notch on both vocal cords in **90%** of cases. The glottic tract was reduced despite the notch in **10%** of cases who presented with slight inspiratory dyspnoea and dysphonia. After 2 repeat post-transverse cordotomies in these 10%, we observed a good glottic tract in all patients at 12ème months.
Our result is comparable to that of **F.I Koné et all** who performed a control nasofibroscopy in all his patients, a good glottic airway was observed in **88.9%** of cases, and 1 case or **11.1%** presented dyspnoea at 3 months. At 6ème, 9ème ,12ème and 14ème months, recovery was good in all patients (2).

CHAPTER V

CONCLUSION

RA is the most feared and classic complication of thyroid surgery. Although it can be transient or permanent, this complication has been described with high rates since the early days of thyroid surgery and was responsible for many deaths. It occurs as a result of injury to the recurrent nerve. The anatomical proximity of the recurrent nerve to the thyroid gland increases the risk of recurrent paralysis. Thanks to standardised surgical techniques, the risk has been reduced but persists. Risk factors for this complication may include:

- Non-recurrent recurrent nerve,
- Nerve attached to the thyroid gland,
- The nerve is located in a fibrous mesh
- The surgeon's experience,
- Thyroid cancer

In Mali, the lack of technical resources is a handicap to patient care. Additional diagnostic tests are complex and not commonly performed in Mali. Treatment of this complication varies depending on whether the RA is unilateral or bilateral. Intraoperatively, prevention involves careful dissection, avoiding excessive traction, and judicious choice of haemostasis techniques and approach to the recurrent nerve. In the case of unilateral RA, the first-line treatment is rehabilitation, as the aim is to re-establish optimal phonation by eliminating false routes, whereas in the case of bilateral RA, the urgent need is to re-establish a sufficient respiratory tract without causing swallowing problems.

RECOMMENDATIONS

At the end of our study, and with a view to contributing to improving the management of ENT disorders, particularly recurrent paralysis, we recommend :

To the health authorities:

- Strengthen the health insurance system to reduce the cost of treating complications.
- Provide hospitals with the equipment they need for stroboscopy and EMG to diagnose and manage RA.
- To provide the ENT department with a fully equipped and functional operating theatre.
- Strengthen ENT staff through training and by recruiting more ENT specialists.
- To facilitate and strengthen the training of doctors specialising in ENT and cervico-facial surgery, both medical and paramedical, qualified in Mali in order to meet needs throughout the country.
- Facilitating the training of specialist anaesthetists.
- Facilitate the training of speech and language therapy specialists.
- Create a postgraduate diploma in thyroid surgery and laryngeal microsurgery.
- To train all those involved in thyroid surgery in the different approaches to the recurrent nerve.

Health agents:

- Dissect the recurrent nerve down to its laryngeal penetration point.
- Mastering techniques for locating the recurrent nerve.
- Adhering to the recommendations for the management of recurrent paralysis is the only way to reduce its morbidity.
- Performing nasofibroscopy or LI pre- and post-operatively
- Organising multidisciplinary care.

To the public:

- All cases of thyroid nodules should be referred early.
- Any case of dysphonia or laryngeal dyspnoea after thyroidectomy should be reported immediately to a doctor.
- Avoid self-medication.

REFERENCES

1. Boukerrous.H, Oussadi. R, La rééducation orthophonique des patients atteints de paralysie récurrentielle unilatérale [Mémoire]. Bejaia: Université Abderrahmane Mira de Bejaia, Faculté des sciences humaines et sociales, Département des sciences sociales, 20192020.89.

2. Kone F I, and Mohamed A K. Post-Thyroidectomy Laryngeal Diplegia in Mali: What Therapeutic Challenge? Exp Rhinol Otolaryngol.2017 1(2). ERO.000508: 24-29. DOI: 10.31031/ERO.2017.01.000508.

3. L. Dbab, L. Adardour, A. Raji, Les paralyses récurrentielles post-thyroïdectomie [These]. Marrakech: Faculty of Medicine and Pharmacy. 2013. 1-3.

4. Les paralyses récurrentielles post-thyroïdectomie [These]. Marrakech: Faculty of Medicine and Pharmacy. 2013. 107.

5. A.-R. Ngo Nyekia, L.-R. Njockb, J. Miloundjac, J.-E. Evehe Vokwelyd, G. Bengonoe . Recurrent laryngeal nerve landmarks during thyroidectomy. European Annals of Otorhinolaryngology, Head and Neck diseases 2015; 132 :265-269.

6. Hung-Chun C,Yu-Cheng P, Tuan-Jen, MDRisk Factors for Thyroid Surgery-Related Unilateral Vocal Fold Paralysis. Laryngoscope.2019; 129 :275-283.

7. Rosato. L, Avenia. N, Bernante. P, et al. Complications of thyroid surgery: analysis of a multicentric study on 14,934 patients operated on in Italy over 5 years. World J Surg 2004;28: 271-6.

8. B. Hammami S. Kallel, N. KolsiI, L. Smaoui, A. Chakroun,I. Charfeddine, A. Ghorbel. Treatment of laryngeal diplegia in closure: contribution of the laser. J. tun ORL. 2011. 26: 37-40.

9. SISSOKO. T. THYROIDECTOMY: REVIEW OF 5 YEARS OF ACTIVITY IN THE DEPARTMENT

D'ORL ET CCF DU CHU GABRIEL TOURE [Thesis in medicine]. Bamako: Faculté de Médecine et d'Odonto-stomatologie; 2018- 2019. 1-115.

10. MEYER. R, STIEN. R. RISQUE VOCAL APRES CHIRURGIE THYROÏDIENNE : PREVENTION ET PRISE EN CHARGE [Dissertation]. Nice: Institut universitaire de la face et du cou; 2020. 1-43.

11. BOUCHET A., GUILLERET J. The larynx. In Bouchet A., Guilleret J. Anatomie topographique et fonctionnelle : le cou - Villeurbanne, SIMEP 1971: 71 - 94.

12. GUERRIER B., BARAZER M. Descriptive, endoscopic and radiological anatomy of the larynx. Encycl. Méd-Chir (Editions Scientifiques et Médicales Elsevier SAS Paris), Oto-rhino-laryngologie, 20-630- A-10,1992: 20.

13. BASTIAN D. The larynx and cervical trachea. In Chevrel J.P. Anatomie clinique : tête et cou - Paris : Springer-verlag 1996 : 341 - 363.

14. CHevalier. D , Dubrulle. F, Vilette. B. Descriptive, endoscopic and radiological anatomy of the larynx. EMC ORL. Paris : ELSEVIER ; 2001.13 [20- 630 - A - 10].

15. BRUGERE J., SCHWAAB G. Squamous cell carcinomas: unity and diversity. In: Brugère Cancers des voies aéro-digestives supérieures. 1st ed. Paris: Flammarion Médecine-Science; 1987:64-8.

16. BEAUVILLAIN De MONTREUIL C. Malignant tumours of the larynx. Rev Prat. 1993; 43 (5) : 631 - 6.

17. EL ANSAR. S. Les cordectomies [Thesis in medicine]. Marrakech: UNIVERSITE CADI AYYAD FACULTE DE MEDECINE ET DE PHARMACIE MARRAKECH; 2021. 1-103.

18. LEHMANN W., PIDOUX J.M. and WIDMANN J.J. The larynx. Microlaryngoscopy and Histopathology. Iharzam Medical, 1978.

19. N.Matar, Remacle.M. Phonosurgery of benign vocal cord tumours. EMC ORL. Paris: ELSEVIER 2018Techniques chirurgicales-Tête et cou. 16.

20. Page. C, Peltier, Strunski. V, Foulon. P, Havet. E et all. Anatomical variation of the inferior laryngeal nerve: application to thyroid surgery. Littérature Scientifique en Santé.

2004 ; 88(281) : 72-72.
21. Kandil. E, Abdelghani. S, Friedlander. P, Alrasheedi. S, Tufano. RP, Bellows. CF, Slakey. D Motor and sensory branching of the recurrent laryngeal nerve in thyroid surgery. Surgery. 2011; 150(6) :1222-7. doi: 10.1016/j.surg.2011.09.002.
22. Zirari. W. Complications of thyroid surgery [Thesis in medicine]. Marrakech: UNIVERSITE CADI AYYAD FACULTE DE MEDECINE ET DE PHARMACIE MARRAKE; 2010.1-179.
23. Jatzko GR, Lisborg PH, Muller MG, Wette VM. Recurrent nerve palsy after thyroid operations: principal nerve identification and a literature review. Surgery. 1994;115:139- 144.
24. Butskiy O, Chang BA, Luu K, McKenzie RM, Anderson DW. A systematic approach to the recurrent laryngeal nerve dissection at the cricothyroid junction. J Otolaryngol Head Neck Surg. 2018; 47-57.
25. Périé S, Aït-Mansour A, Devos M, Sonji G, Baujat B, St Guily JL. Value of recurrent laryngeal nerve monitoring in the operative strategy during total thyroidectomy and parathyroidectomy. Eur Ann Otorhinolaryngol Head Neck Dis. 2013 ;130(3) :131-6.
26. Page C, Cuvelier P, Biet A, Strunski V. Value of intra-operative neuromonitoring of the recurrent laryngeal nerve in total thyroidectomy for benign goitre. The Journal of Laryngology & Otology. 2015 ;129(06) : 553-557.
27. Klopp-Dutote N, Biet-Hornstein A, Guillaume-Souaid G, Strunski V, Page C. Intraoperative neuromonitoring of the vagus nerve during thyroidectomy. A prospective study. Clinical Otolaryngology. 2016;41(5): 454-460;
28. Pardal-Refoyo JL, Ochoa-Sangrador C. Bilateral recurrent laryngeal nerve injury in total thyroidectomy with or without intraoperative neuromonitoring. Systematic review and metaanalysis. Acta OtorrinolaringolEsp. 2016;67:66-7.
29. Al-Qurayshi Z, Kandil E, Randolph GW. Cost-effectiveness of intraoperative nerve monitoring in avoidance of bilateral recurrent laryngeal nerve injury in patients undergoing total thyroidectomy. Br J Surg. 2017;104:1523-1531.
30. Remacle M., Lawson G. Laryngeal paralysis. EMC (Elsevier SAS, Paris), Otolaryngology, 20-675-A-10, 2006.
31. Sanogo. Indications et complications de la laryngectomie totale dans le service ORL et CCF du CHU Gabriel Touré [Thesis]. Bamako: Faculté de médecine et d'odontostomatologie de Bamako; 2021-2022. 1-118.
32. S. Hans, E. de Monès, E. Behm, O. Laccourreye, D. Brasnu . How to perform laryngeal nasofibroscopy in adults? Ann Otolaryngol Chir Cervicofac, 2006; 123, 1, 41-45 © Masson, Paris, 2006.
33. Seddon. H. Surgical disorders of the peripheral nerves second ed. Edinburgh: Churchill Livingston. 1975: 332.
34. Sunderland.S. Nerves and nerves injuries. BJS ; 1969.56 :401-401.
35. Chang Hwan Ryu, Seung Jin Lee, Jae-Gu Cho et al. Care and Management of Voice Change in Thyroid Surgery: Korean Society of Laryngology, Phoniatrics and Logopedics Clinical Practice Guideline. Clinical and Experimental Otorhinolaryngology .2022; 15, (1): 24-48.
36. Lee. JS, Kim. JP, Ryu. JS, Woo. SH. Effect of wound massage on neck discomfort and voice changes after thyroidectomy.ELSEVER.Surgery .2018;164(5):965-71.
37. Stachler. RJ, Francis .DO, Schwartz. SR, Damask .CC, Digoy .GP, Krouse .HJ et al. Clinical practice guideline: hoarseness (dysphonia) (update). American academy of otolaryngology-head and neck surgeryl.2018;158(3): 409-426.
38. Guzman. M, Castro .C, Madrid. S, Olavarria. C, Leiva. M, Munoz. D et al. Air pressure and contact quotient measurements during different semioccluded postures in subjects with different voice conditions.J of voice. 2016 ;30(6) : 759.e1-759.e10.
39. Gabet.C, Spriet.M. Objective and subjective speech therapy analysis of vocal disorders after thyroid surgery [Dissertation]. Amiens (France): Université de Picardie Jules Verne;

2021. 1-98.
40. ARNOUX-SINDT. B, BEUTTER. P, CHEVALIER. D, ORL, DEBRY. C, FUGAIN. C, GIOVANNI. A et al. Adute's recurrent paralysis. Recommendation for clinical practice. SFORL.2022; 1- 11.
41. Remacle.M, Laryngeal paralysis, EMC ORL. Paris: ELMESIER; 2006.35(3): 1-20.
42. Chang Hwan Ryu,Tack-Kyun Kwon ·Heejin Kim ,Han Su Kim4 Jl-Seok Park, Joo Hyun Woo. Guidelines for the Management of Unilateral Vocal Fold Paralysis From the Korean Society of Laryngology, Phoniatrics and Logopedics. Clinical and Experimental Otorhinolaryngology. 2020; 13(4): 340-360.
43. Misron.K, Balasubramanian. A, Irfan.M, Nik F.H.N, Hassan. Bilateral vocal cord palsy post thyroidectomy:lessons learnt [online]. BMJ.2014 (March 2022). 1-3. Available at doi:10.1136/bcr-2013-201033.
44. TEFALI. A. Morbidity of thyroid surgery [Thesis in medicine]. Tlemcen: UNIVERSITE ABOU BEKR BELKAÎD FACULTE DE MEDECINE DR. B. BENZERDJEB - TLEMCEN; 2017-2018. 1-140.
45. N. Christou, M. Mathonnet, What are the complications after total thyroidectomy? Journal of Visceral Surgery (2013) 150, 276-284, Available online at www.sciencedirect.com.
46. Richer SL, Randolph GW. Management of the recurrent laryngeal nerve in thyroid surgery. Op Tech Otolaryngol 2009 ;20:29-34.
47. DM. Hartl , JP.Travagli , S.Leboulleux , E.Baudin , DF.Brasnu , M.Schlumberger . Current concepts in the management of unilateral recurrent laryngeal nerve paralysis after thyroid surgery.N. J Clin Endocrinol Metab.2005 ;90 :3084-8.
48. Sancho.JJ. Risk factors for transient vocal cord palsy after thyroidectomy. Br J Surg 2008;95:961-7.
49. Conessa. CL, SISSOKHO.B, FAYE.M. Les complications de la chirurgie thyroïdienne A L'hopital principal de Dakar A Propos de 155 Interventions. Médecine d'Afrique Noire. 2000 ; 47(3) : 158-160.
50. J.-P. Jeannon, A. A. Orabi, G. A. Bruch, H. A. Abdalsalam, R. Simo. Diagnosis of recurrent laryngeal nerve palsy after thyroidectomy: a systematic review. Journal compilation 2009 Blackwell Publishing Ltd Int J Clin Pract. 2009; 63(4): 624-629.
51. Ouédraogo B.P et al. Goitres in ENT: epidemiological, diagnostic and therapeutic aspects. La revue africaine d'ORL et de chirurgie cervico-faciale 2016; (16) :1-5.
52. Konaté M Etude des goitres bénins dans le service de chirurgie générale et pédiatrique du CHU Gabriel Touré de Bamako à propos de 112 cas. [Thèse]. Mali: FMOS; 2007. 1-109.
53. Renata. MI, Jos. VT a, Sérgio .AR, Elaine. LMT, Regina. HGM. Laryngeal and vocal alterations after thyroidectomy. Brazilian Journal Otorhinolaryngology. 2019 ;85(1) :3-10.
54. Baldé. D, Zounon A.D.S, Ndiaye. C, Adjibabi. W, Yehouessi. B. V. Thyroid Surgery at the ENT Department of the Heinrich Lübké Regional Hospital in Diourbel: 60 Month Review. The journal of medicine and bomedical sciences.2020; 22(4): 1-5.
55. Mok. VM, Oltmann. SC, Chen. H, Sippel. RS, Schneider. DF. Identifying predictors of a difficult thyroidectomy. Journal of Surgical Research. 2014;190:157-63.
56. A. Biet, R. Zaatar, V. Strunski, C. Page. Postoperative complications in total thyroidectomy for Graves' disease: comparison with surgery for non-Basedowian goitres. 2009 Elsevier Masson SAS. Available online at www.sciencedirect.com.
57. ROULET M. La maladie de Basedow : Facteur de risque de complications de la thyroïdectomie totale [Thèse Médecine]. angers (France) : Faculté de santé. Université d'Angers; 2019.1-25.
58. Serpell. JW, Yeung. MJ, Grodski. S. The motor fibers of the recurrent laryngeal nerve are located in the anterior extralaryngeal branch. Ann Surg 2009;249:648-52.
59. Thomas K Chung, MD1, Eben L Rosenthal, MD, FACS1, John R Porterfield, MD, FACS2, William R Carroll, MD, FACS1, Joshua Richman, MD, PhD2, and Mary T Hawn,

MD, FACS21. Examining National Outcomes after Thyroidectomy with Nerve Monitorin. J Am Coll Surg. 2014 ; 219(4) : 765-770g.

APPENDICES

Material Safety Data Sheet

Name: Coulibaly
First name: Assitan kolé
Contact: +22376164166
Email : assitankolec@gmail.com
Title : Epidemiological, diagnostic and therapeutic aspects of post-thyroidectomy recurrent paralysis.
Academic year: 2022-2023
City of defence: Bamako
Country of origin: Mali
Sector of interest: ENT-CCF
Venue: Faculty of Medicine and Odontostomatology (FMOS)

SUMMARY :

Introduction: Recurrent paralysis is dysfunction of one or both of the lower laryngeal nerves, most often resulting in paralysis of the intrinsic muscles of the larynx that are innervated by the lower laryngeal nerves. Post-thyroidectomy recurrent paralysis (RP) is the most frequent and most feared complication.
The aim of our study was to describe the epidemiological, diagnostic and therapeutic aspects of post-thyroidectomy recurrent paralysis.

Methods: This was an observational, descriptive, retrospective study from January 2020 to January 2023.
Our study included patients who had consulted us for dysphonia or dyspnoea after thyroidectomy, or who had consulted us for other laryngeal symptoms after thyroidectomy, and whose nasofibroscopy or suspension laryngoscopy result indicated immobility of one or more vocal cords.

Results: A total of 27 cases were collected. The mean age of our patients was 46.18 years. The most common age range was 41 to 55 years. Females predominated in 96% of cases. Anatomopathological findings did not reveal any signs of malignancy in all patients. Basedow's disease was the main indication for surgery in 51.9% of patients, followed by multi nodular goitre in 40.7%. Total thyroidectomy was performed in 74.1% of patients. We had no information on nerve dissection in 63% of cases. Inspiratory dyspnoea and dysphonia were associated in 81.5% of cases. Laryngeal diplegia accounted for 77.8% and monoplegia for 22.2%. RA was transient in 22.2% and permanent in 77.8%, with a mortality rate of 3.7%. Medical treatment was used in 100% of cases, speech therapy in 77.8% and transverse posterior cordotomy in 95.2%.

Conclusion: In Mali, inadequate technical facilities are a handicap to patient care. Complementary diagnostic tests are complex and not commonly performed in Mali. Treatment of this complication varies depending on whether the RA is unilateral or bilateral.

Key words: thyroidectomy, recurrent nerve, recurrent paralysis, nasofibroscopy, posterior transverse cordotomy, ENT-CCF.

SUMMARY :

Background : Recurrent paralysis is the dysfunction of one or both lower

laryngeal nerves, most often resulting in paralysis of the intrinsic muscles of the larynx which are innervated by the lower laryngeal nerves. Post-thyroidectomy recurrent paralysis (PR) is the most common and feared complication.
The objective of our study was to describe the epidemiological, diagnostic and therapeutic aspects of post-thyroidectomy recurrent paralysis.
Material and Methods: This was an observational, descriptive and retrospective study spanning from January 2020 to January 2023.
Patients who consulted for dysphonia or dyspnea after thyroidectomy were included in our study; who consulted for other laryngeal symptoms after a thyroidectomy and whose result of nasofibroscopy or suspension laryngoscopy concluded that one or more vocal cords were immobility.
Results : In total we collected 27 cases. The average age of our patients was 46.18 years. The most represented age group was 41 to 55 years. We noted a female predominance in 96%. The anatomo-pathological result did not find signs of malignancy in all patients. Graves' disease was the main indication for surgery in 51.9% followed by multi-nodular goiter in 40.7%. Total thyroidectomy was performed in 74.1%. We had no information on nerve dissection in 63%. Inspiratory dyspnea and dysphonia were associated in 81.5%. Laryngeal diplegia accounted for 77.8% and monoplegia in 22.2%.%. PR was transient in 22.2%, permanent in 77.8% including a mortality rate of 3.7%. Medical treatment in 100% of cases, speech therapy in 77.8% and posterior transverse cordotomy was performed in 95.2%.
Conclusion : In Mali, the insufficiency of the technical platform constitutes a handicap in the care of patients. Additional diagnostic examinations are complex and are not common practice in Mali. The treatment of this complication varies depending on whether it is unilateral or bilateral RA.
Keywords: thyroidectomy, recurrent nerve, recurrent paralysis, nasofibroscopy, Posterior cordotomy, ORL-CCF.

FACT SHEET :

Epidemiological, diagnostic and therapeutic aspects of post-thyroidectomy recurrent paralysis.

File no.

Sampling date

1-IDENTIFICATION

Surname and first name Sex

Age (years) Address: Tel

------------ - - - ------. Profession :

2- ANTECEDENTS AND LIFESTYLE :

-Medical: -diabetes: no /...... / yes /...... / -HTA: no /...... / yes/...... / -Asthma: no /...... / yes /...... / -Sickle cell disease: no /...... / yes /...... / -laryngeal pathology: no /...... / yes /...... / which .... -HIV : no /...... / yes /...... / - Surgical: - ENT surgery: no /...... / yes /...... / which .... -Other surgery: no /...... / yes /...... / which .... -alcohol: no /...... / yes /...... / -smoking: no /...... / yes /...... /

3-RECRUITMENT METHOD :

Emergency / /Consultation box / / refer / /

4 GENERAL EXAMINATION OF THE PATIENT :

Patient's general condition according to the WHO: Consciousness : Conjunctivo-palmo-plantar staining :

BP : T° : Pulse: IMO :

FR :

5- ORAL PHYSICAL EXAMINATION :

1-Examination of the oral cavity and oropharynx

2-Skin and face test :

3-Otoscopy :

4-Rhinoscopy :

5-Examination of lymph nodes :

6-PREOPERATIVE LARYNGEAL ANATOMY :

-Functional signs: Absent /...... / Laryngeal dyspnoea /...... / Dysphonia /...... / Swallowing problems /...... / Other:..................... -Duration of symptoms: .... -Nasofibroscopy: not performed /...... / Pharyngo-laryngeal morphology: ....
....

7-CHARACTERISTICS OF THE DISEASE THROID OPERATED :

Modular goitre /...... / Diffuse goitre /...... / Hypothyroidism /...... / Hyperthyroidism /...... / Compressive goitre /...... / Plunging goitre /...... /

Definitive histopathological diagnosis (malignancy)
....

8-SURGICAL REMOVAL :

- The surgeon: ENT surgeon /...... / Other surgeons :............ - Intubation: easy /...... / difficult /...... / unknown /...... / - Operative procedure: -Total thyroidectomy /...... / -Lobo-isthmectomy: right /...... / left /...... / -Node drainage: no /...... / right /...... / left /...... / Bilateral /...... / Type :..............................

-Dissection of recurrent nerve: no /...... / yes /...... / neurostimulation /...... / nerve damage /......../ unknown/...... /

9- POST-OPERATION :

Simple /...... / haematoma /...... / superinfection /...... / Hypo-parathyroid /...... / resuscitation /...... / -Dyspnoea: inspiratory /...... / expiratory /...... / Staging of dyspnoea according to Chevalier Jackson and Pineau: ....
Time to onset after surgery: .... -Dysphonia: Hoarse voice /...... / bitonal /...... / fatigable /...... / Time to onset: .... -Deglutination disorder: Type:............................
Time to onset:............................... -length of hospital stay:.....................................
- **Nasofibroscopy**: -Right vocal cord: Mobility normal /...... / Immobile/...... / Hypokinesia /...... / Position: median /...... / paramedian /...... / intermediate /...... / abduction /...... / Tone: normal /...... / hypotonia /...... / -Left vocal cord: Mobility normal /...... / Immobile /...... / Hypokinesia /...... / Position: median /...... / paramedian /...... / intermediate /...... / abduction /...... / Tone: normal /...... / hypotonia /...... / -Rightrytenoid: Position: normal /...... / abnormal /...... / Mobility on coughing: mobile /...... / fixed /...... / -Left **atenoid**: Position: normal /...... / abnormal /...... / Mobility on cough: mobile /...... / fixed /...... / - Laryngeal diplegia /...... /

10- MANAGEMENT OF PARALYSIS RECURRENCE :

1- Medical: -Corticoid: injectable /...... / VO /...... / aerosol /...... / -ATB: injectable /...... / VO /...... / 2-Surgical: Tracheotomy /...... / posterior cordotomy /...... / Date of operation:................................ 3- Speech rehabilitation

-Deadline for completion:...................... -Number of sessions:........................

11-EVOLUTON :

-AT 3 MONTHS :

Clinical manifestations: no /...... / dyspnoea /...... / dysphonia /...... / dysphagia /...... / cough /...... / On follow-up nasofibroscopy:
....
....
....

- AT 6 MONTHS :

Clinical manifestations: no /...... / dyspnoea /...... / dysphonia /...... / dysphagia /...... / cough /...... / On follow-up nasofibroscopy:
....
....

....
-AT 9 MONTHS :
Clinical manifestations: no /...... / dyspnoea /...... / dysphonia /...... / dysphagia /...... / cough /...... / On follow-up nasofibroscopy:
....
....
....
- 12 MONTHS :
Clinical manifestations: no /...... / dyspnoea /...... / dysphonia /...... / dysphagia /...... / cough /...... / On follow-up nasofibroscopy:
....
....
....
Revision of posterior transverse cordotomy: no /...... / number of times.........................

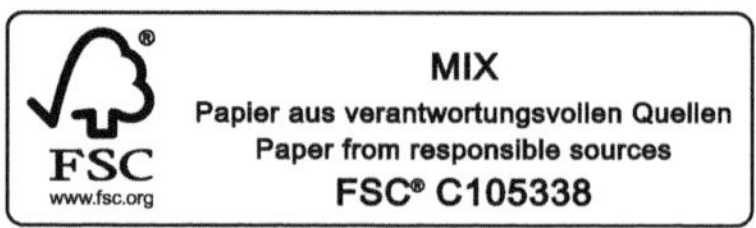

Printed by Books on Demand GmbH, Norderstedt / Germany